frédéric
Fekkai

CLARKSON POTTER/PUBLISHERS
NEW YORK

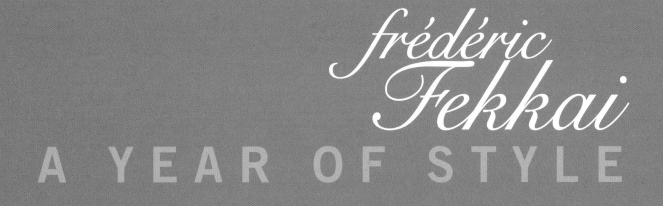

frédéric Fekkai
A YEAR OF STYLE

PHOTOGRAPHS BY TARA SGROI

DEDICATION

I dedicate this book to my many loyal clients and staff members, in both the New York and Los Angeles salons, who share my love of creativity and appetite for beauty, style, and life.

To my mother Anna Maria, my son Alexandre, and E.R.J. for the love and passion for life we share.

Published by Clarkson Potter/Publishers, New York
Member of the Crown Publishing Group
Random House, Inc. New York, Toronto, London, Sydney, Auckland
www.randomhouse.com

CLARKSON N. POTTER is a trademark and POTTER and colophon are registered trademarks of Random House, Inc.

Printed in Japan

Design by Richard Ferretti

Library of Congress Cataloging-in-Publication Data
Fekkai, Frédéric.
    A year of style / by Frédéric Fekkai.
    1. Fashion. 2. Clothing and dress. 3. Beauty, Personal. 4. Women—Health and hygiene. I. Title.
TT507.F43 2000
646'.34—dc21   99-086764

ISBN 0-609-60503-8

10 9 8 7 6 5 4 3 2 1
First Edition

ACKNOWLEDGMENTS

I would like to give special thanks and acknowledgment to my collaborative team, especially Noel Robinson, Simonetta Morrison, Kimberly Callet, and Caroline Keavy, who have contributed a great deal of work and love to make *A Year of Style* helpful and fun!

Thank you to Tara Sgroi, who has captured the essence of style, humor, and simplicity of life through her camera lens. To Troy Word, an amazing photographer, for shooting the cover. And to fellow photographers Oberto Gili, Bruno Gaget, Anne Shea Buckingham, Henri Del Olmo, Regan Cameron, Jean-Jacques L'Heritier, Corbis Images, Tony Stone Photography, and Encre Noire. To Véronique Vienne, who is not only a marvelous writer, but a person who can relate to and understand casual chic. Jean Godfrey June. To the many models, modeling agencies, stylists, makeup artists and hair designers including Melissa Keller, Manda Garcia, Greet Germis, Corine Russel, Shannon Shultz, Mieke Meulman, Silvana Krijger, Marilyn Sieler, Claudia Wagner, Margriet Wever, Alexandra Redmer, Nathalie Lyon, Aurielie Claudel, An Hayward, Amanda Dzwil, Tiffany Johnson, Alina Vacariu, Roseanne Repetti, Victor Caetano, Yvonne Frowein, Lucy Sykes, Marie Josee LaFontaine, Racine Christensen, Michael Aleman, and Fabrice Gili.

Hilary Swank, Gillian Anderson, Salma Hayek, Mira Sorvino, Courteney Cox Arquette, Brooke Shields, Liv Tyler.

Suzie McKenzie, Stephanie Sider, Daniel Jouve, Gil Dez, Charlie de Montemarco, Michel Jean, and all my dear friends in Aix-en-Provence.

Also, thanks to Richard Ferretti, and to the entire team at Clarkson Potter: Mark McCauslin, Jane Treuhaft, and Jane Searle. To Pam Krauss, my editor, who believed in *A Year of Style* and made it happen. She has been instrumental in putting this book together, and I love *her* style.

CONTENTS

INTRODUCTION

Natural. Effortless. Chic. These words are music to my ears. They evoke the very essence of a style that's both simple and elegant. I believe that if you know how to be simple—with your hair, your makeup, your clothes, your lifestyle—you can do anything you want, and never go wrong.

Style is not about age, or height, or weight—it's about a sense of ease, a sense of dignity, and a sense of individuality shining through. The elegant women of my childhood in Provence would dress and style themselves the same way, whether they were young or old. Simplicity is the key to that style, that effortless chic.

So, if I had to describe this book, I would say it's a month-by-month guide to simplicity. But simplicity, of course, is not as easy as it sounds. Take Picasso, for instance. At the end of his life, his work was simple, almost childlike. He could never have done what he did, though, without his classical training, which taught him to observe nature and draw from it. It is the same thing with style. First you have to learn to observe. To notice details. To interpret what you see.

I learned to observe by sitting at the terrace of the famous Deux Garçons café in Aix-en-Provence, my hometown in the South of France. Because Aix is a small yet spirited city, watching its street life is a fascinating spectacle. To this day, I am still spellbound by its colors, its movements, and its sounds—and by the way the beautiful sunlight exalts the shape and texture of almost everything.

I often wondered why Aix is considered one of the most style-conscious towns in France. Is it its glorious medieval past? Its superb 17th- and 18th-century architecture? Its intellectual life centered around its chic university? Its famous music festival?

Keep guessing. Though Aix richly deserves its ten pages in the Michelin guide, there is more to it than just sightseeing. Recently, I came to the conclusion that Aix is unique because, though sophisticated, the town is not alienated from nature.

Sunshine, tall trees, flowers, and countless fountains babbling on shaded squares bring nature right into the heart of this busy city. At every turn, century-old plane trees line up the avenues. Its main street, the famous Cours Mirabeau, has no less than four rows of these gigantic trees. Ancient fountains in the middle of the street slow down traffic. In the dappled light of this majestic boulevard—a green tunnel, really—people wander up and down the wide sidewalks. To take in the sights and enjoy the serenity of this natural setting, they eventually stop at one of the many terrace cafés, where they linger for hours in front of a *citron pressé* or a pastis.

The appreciation of nature teaches us to have style because it gives us a gentler, wiser, and more poetic view of the world. I noticed that men and women who have style are often people who are in contact with nature. It never fails: In the course of a casual conversation with some quietly stylish people, I usually discover that they are passionate about gardening, sailing, or horse breeding—or that they are experts in forestry, landscaping, geology, kayaking, rock climbing, flower arrangements, you name it.

Last summer, I was introduced to a wealthy man who lives part of the year in Saint-Tropez. We began to chat, and he took me outside to show me his field of olive trees. Proudly, he began to explain to me in great detail how his trees establish their root system, why their wood is resistant to decay, and when is the best time to harvest their olives. While he spoke, I was watching him: He wore light canvas slacks, a blue plaid cotton shirt, a pair of espadrilles, and a straw hat. There was not a single designer label or brand name on his clothes. I suddenly realized that he had incredible style, not because he was wealthy and could afford to dress well, but because he cared about his trees.

Simply put, this is the ultimate secret of style: Be natural. Don't go against nature—your nature. Don't deny it—work with it. You cannot force things to be what they aren't. From the way you smile to the way you walk, dress, eat, or talk, be authentic. Stay away from what's artificial. I know for a fact that, even more than so-called good taste, what you need to have style is a nature-inspired and unpretentious way of looking at things.

A YEAR'S WORTH OF STYLE

Style is natural but never static. In this book, chapters go month by month, and the calendar moves day by day, to reflect the spirit of the kind of adjustments that will keep your personal style fresh and alive. I suggest you welcome each new season with a ritual of your own. Make bouquets of seasonal flowers. Reorganize your closet. Throw away old shoes. Buy a new lipstick. Eat vegetables grown locally. Take a slow drive down your favorite country road.

In Provence, people eat food and wear clothes that celebrate the season—and by the season I mean the specific month. The cherries for clafoutis are incredible in June—sweet, sour, tingling with flavor, so that's when we eat them. In the heat of August, the linen sundresses and the cotton scarves come out, in colors—deep coral reds, rich cerulean blue—that stand up to the heat, that mimic its intensity.

I'd watch the women at the farmers' markets every week, and marvel at the little adjustments they made as the seasons came and went: A young girl who always put her hair up with a pair of chopsticks during the summer would use a pencil instead, once school started. The elegant mother of four who went everywhere with a huge, chic leather bag would change to a straw panier as summer approached. The man in my mother's favorite antique shop changed from thin khakis to jeans to corduroys as the Provençal winds got harsher and colder. The flowers at our favorite café changed every day: poppies, lavender, lilies.

Life is different now, in that we all travel everywhere, at any time of year. So the adjustments we make have to be quicker: You might have a two-week business trip that goes from Dallas to Seattle to Brussels to Miami. Fashion trends change faster, too. The key to staying stylish in the face of all these demands on your wardrobe and your schedule is to accentuate what's best about you. Instead of trying to keep up with the latest fashion, pick only the changes you like and have a ball.

Underneath it all, there needs to be a core of simplicity and even practicality behind those choices. Style is a few great things you can always depend on, from a slipdress that never fails to make you feel sexier and a pair of sunglasses that simply oozes sophistication and glamour, to lavender water sprayed on your sheets and pillow cases to make you sleep like a baby, to a recipe that instantly charms your guests. Remember: Style is just another word for what makes you feel better and what makes your life easier, month after month.

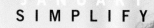

JANUARY
SIMPLIFY

GET A GREAT DATE PLANNER.
PICK ONE WITH A BEAUTIFUL
COVER, SINCE YOU'LL BE
LOOKING AT IT EVERY DAY.

SCHEDULE A FACIAL TO
REVIVE YOUR COMPLEXION
AFTER HOLIDAY EXCESSES.

**MAKE HOT CHOCOLATE THE
FRENCH WAY:** BREAK A SWISS
CHOCOLATE BAR IN SQUARES.
MELT THEM IN A SAUCEPAN
ON LOW HEAT. ADD WHOLE
MILK SLOWLY WHILE STIRRING.
SIMMER GENTLY FOR FIVE
MINUTES. WHISK BEFORE
SERVING.

Your New Year's resolution is to take more time for yourself, isn't it? So start by cutting away what's not essential. Simplify things. January is a great month for less-is-more makeovers: style adjustments that allow you to spend less time in front of the mirror, but more time feeling wonderful.

The kind of transformation I have in mind has nothing to do with before-after pictures in magazines. No one is interested in superficial cosmetic fixes that last only a few days. What you need is long-term thinking: There are no fewer than 365 days in a year, and you need an approach to personal style that is versatile enough, easy enough, to work for every one of them.

Be creative, be confident. A closet with only ten items in it can be stronger than one with hundreds. A beautiful woman I remember in Aix-en-Provence always wore the same scarf—wrapped around her head when she was driving, at her throat under a white raincoat, around her waist as a sarong in the late summer. She clearly loved it and it suited her, so why have a dozen? It's that sort of gesture that reflects real style.

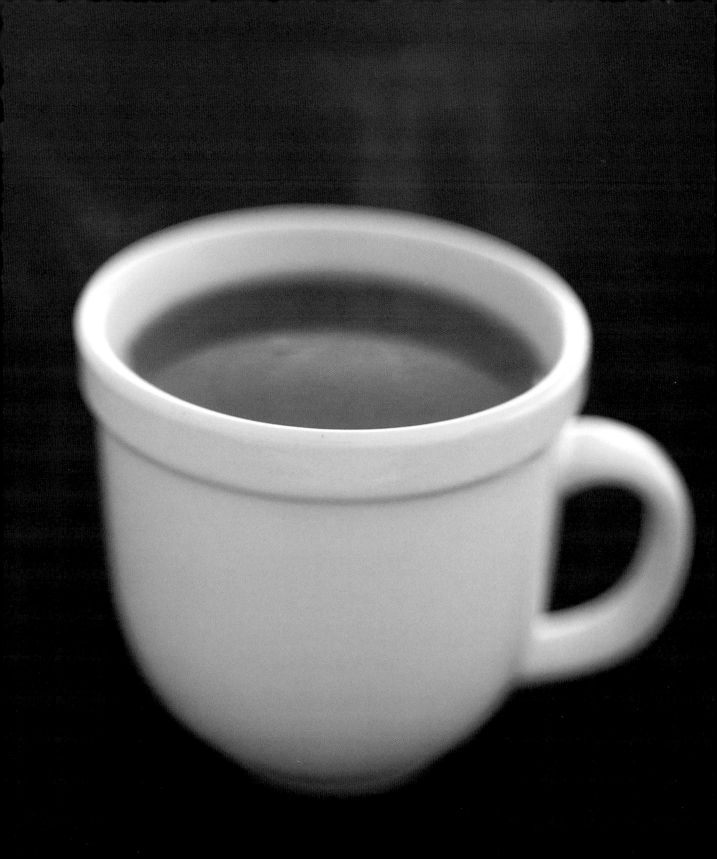

NOW THAT THE HOLIDAY CROWDS ARE GONE, **GO SHOPPING.** BUY A NEW COAT AND SOME GREAT BOOTS ON SALE. NOTHING LIFTS THE SPIRITS LIKE A BARGAIN.

MAKE YOUR OWN BREAD. NOTHING TASTES BETTER.

LEARN TO SIT PROPERLY, FEET FLAT ON THE FLOOR, WITH YOUR CHIN PULLED SLIGHTLY TOWARD YOUR NECK TO ELONGATE YOUR SPINE.

Are you spending an hour every day styling your hair? You need a new cut. Are your nails brittle, your cuticles dry? Take a break from the major manicures and focus on moisturizing oils, luxurious creams. Have your nails buffed instead of polished.

When my clients come to me with questions, doubts, issues, hesitations, and anxieties, I suggest we back up. "Let's not make it more complicated than it already is," I tell them. "Let's not blame whomever or whatever for your color or cut problems. You are an attractive woman, don't worry—you just have to know what to do to enhance your own beauty, subtly."

Therein lies the secret of my success—I eliminate problems. I create a look that fits like a glove because it works with the givens of your life—the shape of your face, your coloring, your lifestyle—rather than imposing a style on them. The elements of your own personal style are already there; all I do is put the last piece of the beauty puzzle in place. I don't change a look for the sake of change or for my ego. I just finish the picture.

My real pleasure is subtracting, not adding. I like to eliminate, to bring out the shine by refining and polishing a look. But first I have to help a client unlearn everything she thinks she knows. For example, before I cut hair, we sit down and talk for a while. We discuss her beauty dilemmas in an orderly fashion. I have a few simple questions I ask her to find out what she thinks her main problem is:

✳ **Texture?** ✳ **Shine?** ✳ **Length?** ✳ **Volume?** ✳ **Shape?** ✳ **Color?**

Only after she answers these questions can I start making changes. No fuss. No long list of directions. I just tell her what not to do, which is easy to remember. I make very simple recommendations, from what products to use and how, to a few do's and don'ts for styling that are easy to remember.

FINDING—
AND INTERVIEWING—
A STYLIST

It seems obvious, but it's crucial: Who do you know whose hair looks fabulous? Ask them where (and to whom) they go. Don't immediately go for a cut, take it slower. Book a blow-dry with the stylist you're thinking of. You can ask, if you were to cut my hair, what would you do? Once you've set aside the time for a real consultation, here are some key questions to ask yourself as you talk to your stylist:

∗ DO YOU FEEL COMFORTABLE with the stylist? You should like his or her sense of style, meaning clothing, grooming, personality, everything.

∗ IS THE STYLIST ASKING YOU questions, giving ideas and suggestions that relate to your personality, rather than pointing to a style on the wall or in a book?

∗ IS THE STYLIST ADDRESSING the health of your hair, not just proposing to cut off split ends? The two of you should be talking about conditioners and rinses that enhance shine and bounce, and special treatments that can prevent or repair damage due to the environment, such as pollution, sun, chlorine, humidity, or dry air.

∗ ONCE YOU'VE AGREED ON A LOOK, does the stylist preview how you'll need to blow it dry, wash it, maintain it? These are all things to think about before actually getting the cut.

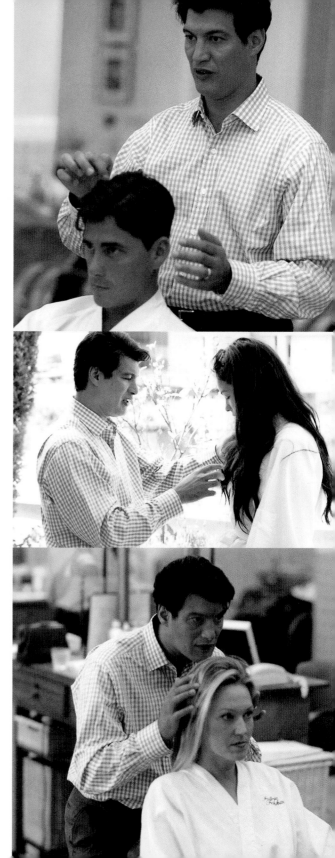

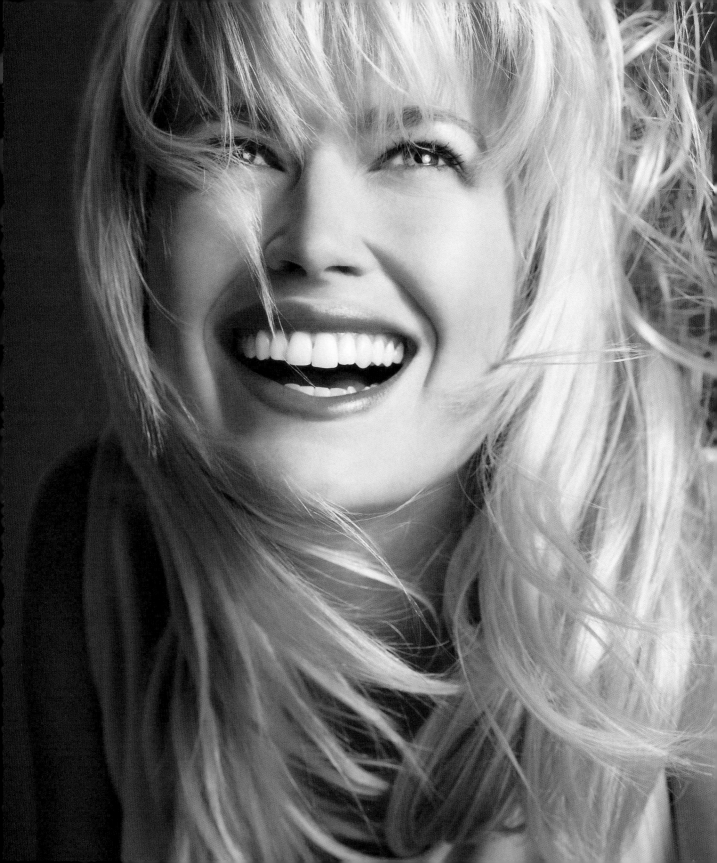

STYLE
IT'S KNOWING WHAT NOT TO DO

As a young man living and working in Provence and later Paris, my aesthetic sensibility was shaped by the kind of effortless elegance that seems to be second nature to so many French women. When clients ask me what they should be doing to improve their look I invariably say: Less! The fundamentals of modern, fresh, uncontrived style are quite basic: Clean, shiny hair. Clear skin. Not too much makeup. Very little jewelry, only what's needed to create a sense of balance. Follow these recommendations and you can't go wrong.

It's human nature, though, to want a more detailed road map to beauty, and every day I get questions from clients wanting hints on perfecting their look. I'm happy to oblige—I've never been shy about voicing my opinions— but rather than try to explain what to do, I prefer to tell people what *not* to do. Indeed, the wrong note can spoil the most elegant scheme and turn an otherwise beautiful woman into an ordinary one. Here are some of the most common mistakes I see:

* **Too much foundation**
* **Harsh lipstick**
* **Obvious lip contour**
* **Heavy eye makeup**
* **Cheap or generic-looking accessories**
* **Too much hairspray**
* **Overdone highlights or overprocessed hair**
* **Artificial-looking nails**

RENEW FRIENDSHIPS. SCHEDULE LUNCH WITH SOMEONE YOU HAVEN'T SEEN FOR A WHILE.

GET AN ANTI-COLD-FINGERS PARAFFIN MANICURE. THE HEAT FROM THIS TREATMENT OPENS UP YOUR PORES AND ENCOURAGES BLOOD CIRCULATION.

START A JOURNAL. RECORD YOUR THOUGHTS AND ACCOMPLISHMENTS. GET TO KNOW YOURSELF.

HAVE A SELF-TANNING TREATMENT. PRETEND YOU HAVE JUST BEEN TO THE CARIBBEAN.

IN THE WORLD OF E-MAIL AND FAXES, IT'S STILL MORE CHIC TO HANDWRITE THANK-YOU NOTES TO FRIENDS AND FAMILY FOR GIFTS RECEIVED AND PARTIES ATTENDED OVER THE HOLIDAYS.

ARE YOU WEARING A HAT? IT SHOULD MATCH THE COLOR OF YOUR COAT— OR YOUR SHOES.

STYLE "DON'TS"

These style lapses are not my clients' fault, but do reflect the desire we all have to fit ourselves into a prevailing notion of beauty, regardless of our own personal style. Sadly, that kind of contrived beauty never looks natural, and unnatural is not modern. Period. So . . .

1 **DON'T ASSUME THERE IS SOMETHING WRONG WITH YOU.** If your hairdresser tells you that your hair is too thin, too thick, too flat, too straight, too curly, you have the wrong hairdresser. It's like a doctor telling you that you can't get well because you are sick.

2 **DON'T BE AFRAID TO BE CLASSIC.** Many women say to me, "I don't want anything classic," assuming classic equals boring. With all due respect, they don't know what they are talking about. Classic in my view can be very fashionable, and if a look fits you, whether it's classic or not, it's cool. Anna Wintour (editor-in-chief of *Vogue* magazine), for instance, has a flawless signature style based on a classic bob; year in, year out she looks of the moment. She is cool.

3 **DON'T TRY TO LOOK LIKE EVERYONE ELSE.** Having a signature hairstyle can be very effective—dare I mention Donald Trump, Meg Ryan, Cher. Changing your hairstyle often can also work if you keep your own personality and identity. I love to see artists like Madonna or David Bowie reinventing themselves at each new album launch. But changing your look to follow every trend just shows insecurity.

4 **DON'T GO TOO BLOND.** I hate to see beautiful women with over-bleached hair. When you bleach your hair too much, the hair becomes porous and loses its natural shine. Eventually it will begin to look coarse and dull. I strongly suggest weaving your own natural hair color into the look.

5 DON'T GLITTER. Tone down over-the-top highlights, make your hair darker and richer, almost the color of blond tobacco. While you are at it, take off most of your gold jewelry and lose the glitzy nail polish.

6 DON'T ADOPT A REGIONAL LOOK. If you live in a part of the country where women are expected to sport long bleached blond hair, heavy eyeliner, and cheap-looking clothes, pack your bags and move! If you live in a neighborhood where permanent tattoos, long square nails, and pierced navels are considered hip, change zip codes! I see so many beautiful women who style themselves according to the community not their personality. For that reason alone they look older and matronly or cheap and ordinary.

7 DON'T HIDE YOUR CHARACTER. Too many women try to hide their real character in order to appear more "feminine." It's such a shame. Femininity is a balance between curves and angles—between the curve of the brows and the angle of the jawline, or between the curve of the cheekbones and the angle of the haircut. The most beautiful women are both hard and soft, straightforward and mysterious, confident and kind.

8 DON'T BE TOO SERIOUS. Accessories are a perfect way to express your state of mind and flaunt your attitude. Find a pair of shoes and a great handbag to enhance your feminity *and* your humor—it should be fun.

9 DON'T TRY TO LOOK PICTURE-PERFECT. By being completely correct, you are always a little wrong.

MAKE YOURSELF A CAFÉ AU LAIT. MIX STRONG COFFEE AND HEATED MILK IN A DEEP BOWL, ONE-THIRD COFFEE TO TWO-THIRDS MILK.

APPLY A DROP OF VITAMIN E TO YOUR SKIN BEFORE YOUR MOISTURIZER TO PROTECT YOUR FACE ALL DAY LONG FROM THE DRYING EFFECT OF COLD AIR AND HEAT.

PLAN A PAJAMA PARTY FOR ONE: RENT A GREAT CLASSIC MOVIE. SLIP INTO A PAIR OF PALE BLUE FLANNEL PAJAMAS. SETTLE INTO BED WITH A TRAY TABLE WHILE YOU WATCH THE MOVIE.

MAKE A COMMITMENT TO
BEAUTIFUL NAILS. SCHEDULE
A WEEKLY MANICURE
APPOINTMENT.

*How the wit
brightens! How
the style refines!*
—ALEXANDER POPE

OUT WITH THE OLD, IN
WITH THE NEW: THROW
OUT YOUR MASCARA AND
BUY A NEW ONE.

SIMPLIFY
YOUR LOOK

The best way to start the new year is to get rid of last year. Last year is that jumble of old lipsticks at the bottom of your bag. It's that complicated skin-care regimen you always avoid. It's that trendy color that didn't really flatter you. It's that pale-colored wrap that seems to collect dirt.

Your makeup bag is a crucial spot on which to focus your simplifying efforts. Women are forever coming into my salon and opening up their makeup bags in utter desperation; the problem is nearly always that they're carrying around too much stuff: Do you really need six shades of lipstick? What about all those eye shadow compacts? Simplifying your makeup routine will do wonders for your look.

One of the smartest-looking women I know carries nothing in her bag but a single, sheer lip stain, which she uses as blush, highlighter, and gloss. If she's going out, she applies more of it, for a more dramatic look. While this kind of minimalism isn't for everyone, the idea of it—that confidence, that verve, that style—most certainly is.

RIGHT: YOU DON'T NEED A LOT OF MAKEUP TO LOOK "FINISHED."
A GROOMED BROW AND RICH LIPS LOOK GREAT ON PALE SKIN
WITH DARK HAIR. THE HAIR IS SIMPLE TOO: LONG HAIR ALL ONE
LENGTH EXCEPT TO THE SIDE, WHERE IT'S ANGLED FROM THE
CHEEKBONES TO THE BOTTOM.

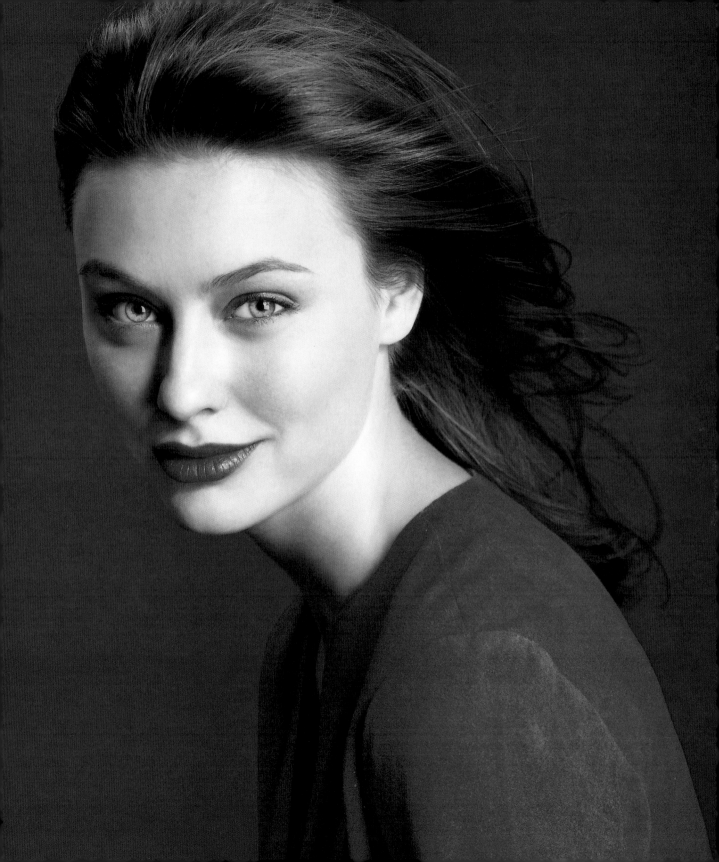

**SPEND AN EVENING
STARTING A NEW FAMILY
ALBUM.** FIND ONE OR TWO
PHOTOGRAPHS WORTH
DISPLAYING IN REALLY
SPECIAL FRAMES.

LEARN YOUR GEOGRAPHY.
IT'S EMBARRASSING NOT TO
KNOW WHERE TIBET IS
LOCATED.

BUY NEW SHEETS, WITH A
TOUCH OF WARM COLORS,
TO REMIND YOU OF SUMMER.

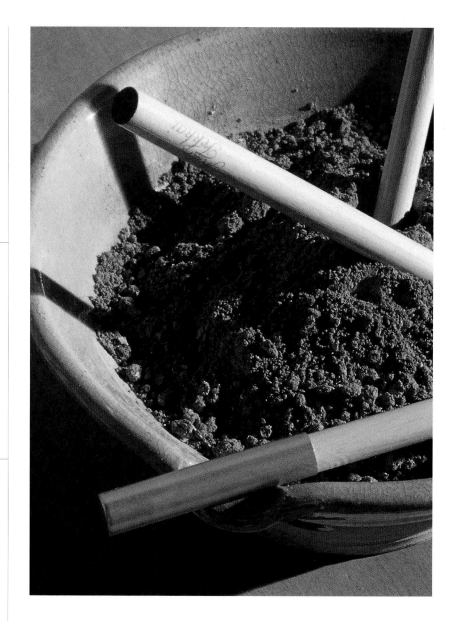

Makeup isn't a mask to hide behind, it's a bit of something wonderful that tweaks the way you look and makes you feel drop-dead gorgeous. It should be fun, easy, and above all, natural.

* **FIRST APPLY SUNSCREEN**, at least SPF 15, every day, without exception.
* **UNLESS YOUR SKIN IS OILY**, apply a little bit of moisturizer. It will allow foundation to go on smoothly, and leave your skin with a natural sheen.
* **STIPPLE CONCEALER** on barely noticeable imperfections: tiny lesions, small scars, liver spots, broken blood vessels, etc. Unlike some foundations, a good concealer will not emphasize fine lines and creases, as long as you use a small stiff brush and apply it in repeated touches. Then blend in with a finger. It works wonders—your face will look almost "airbrushed."
* **DAB A LITTLE MORE CONCEALER** on the area between your eyes, on both sides of the bridge of your nose. It will erase dark circles or shadows.
* **AFTER CONCEALER**, you will need very little foundation, if any. Apply at the center of your face and blend outward. Don't cover your face.
* **USE BARELY VISIBLE EYE SHADOW**, and never match your shadow to your clothing just to coordinate colors.
* **APPLY ONLY ONE COAT OF MASCARA**. To avoid clumping, turn your brush against your lashes while applying.
* **POWDER ONLY IF**, when, and where you need it, and always with a big fat brush: (1) on your cheekbones for a hint of color, (2) on your nose to minimize highlights, (3) on your jawline to emphasize its contour.
* **POLISH YOUR LIPS** with a coat of yummy lipstick. But don't choose a shocking color that's so outrageous it will take away from other beautiful features. You want people to remember your face, not the color of your lipstick.

Now take the rest of your makeup—the eyeliners, the lip liners, the brow pencils, the lip glosses, the glitzy eye shadows, the highlighting dust, and the pile of lipsticks you save for very special occasions—and pack it all in a pretty box. If you can live without the box for the next month, dump the whole thing.

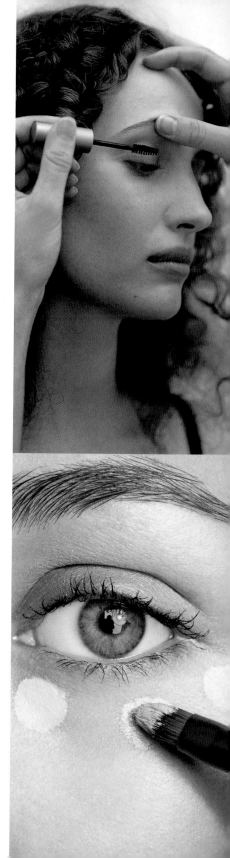

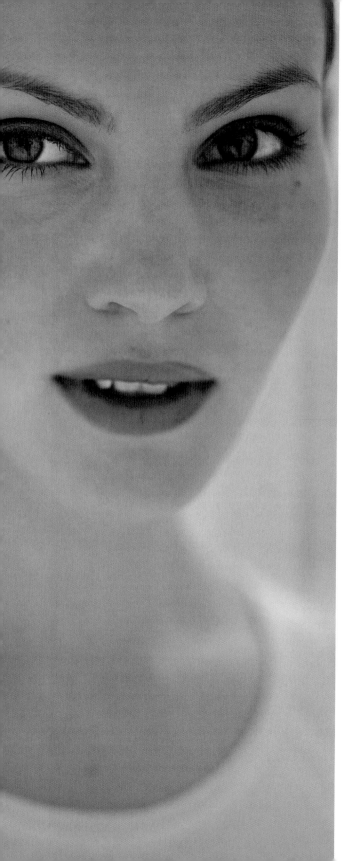

THE NATURAL FACE

This face is refreshingly appealing and looks great on most women.

EYES Stick with two shades of neutral shadow for the eyes (pencil is just too harsh for this look). The first shade should be very subtle and sheer; apply it across the lid, up to the brow bone in order to highlight the entire eye. The second shade should be a deeper nude shadow to even out the skin tone over the lid. If you can't leave the house without mascara, just a quick swipe will give you enough lash definition to finish off this soft eye.

CHEEKS Stick with a rose blush for fresh appeal (especially if you have fair skin). Apply the blush on the apple of the cheeks, judiciously.

LIPS Again, the rose tones are also the place to look for lip colors. Stay away from any thick, matte colors and choose something with a little gloss to it (though not metallic—too obvious). You can also apply just a layer of gloss over your favorite deep rose lipstick.

NAILS A sheer, clean wash of pink or another pale neutral gives a well-manicured yet totally natural finish to this modern look.

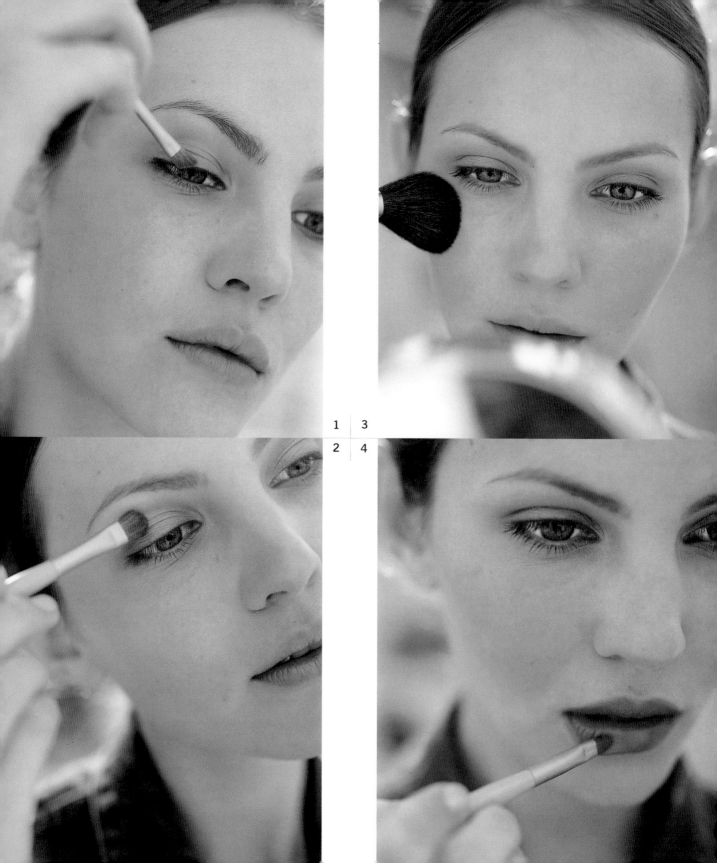

1 | 3
2 | 4

PUT YOUR TO-DO LIST IN A VISIBLE PLACE. AS YOU CROSS OFF TASKS YOU'LL SEE HOW MUCH YOU GET DONE.

TREAT CHAPPED HANDS BEFORE GOING TO SLEEP BY RUBBING THEM WITH RICH MOISTURIZING CREAM AND SLIPPING ON COTTON GLOVES. WAKE UP WITH DELIGHTFULLY SMOOTH SKIN.

PAINT THE INSIDE OF YOUR CLOSET A FAVORITE COLOR— OR DO AS THEY DO IN PROVENCE AND UPHOLSTER IT IN FABRIC. IT'S A HIDDEN LUXURY THAT WILL MAKE YOU SMILE EVERY TIME YOU OPEN THE DOOR.

EYEBROW IMPACT

Eyebrows contribute to the overall harmony of your face while emphasizing the most lively side of your personality. But getting your brows right can be tricky: You need someone to look at them from all sides, just as you need someone to stand back to tell you if a painting is hanging properly. That's why you should start off with a professional shaping and go back every other month or so to keep the line clean and true; afterwards, keep your brows neat and polished between visits by tweezing on your own.

THE CURVE OF THE BROWS helps balance the lines and angles of your face (and your haircut). The standard arch rises ¾ inch from the starting point and falls ¼ inch below that point at the end. If you have a round face, a more pronounced angle will offset the roundness; a more rounded arch will soften a long or angular face.

PLUCK INSTEAD OF WAXING. The wear and tear on your skin of waxing can cause longterm damage. The eye area contains some of the most sensitive muscles in your body, so treat them gently.

TO ADD DEFINITION to your brows, brush your eyebrows straight up, then smooth the top of the arch. Fill in as needed with light eyebrow pencil strokes, blending with a short brush. Never draw above your natural brow line.

DON'T TRY TO STAIN OR DYE your eyebrows the same color as your hair. It never works: The texture of brow hair is not the same as the texture of your hair, so the color won't take in the same way.

NEVER TATTOO YOUR BROWS. All my clients who do always come to regret it when they want to change their hairstyle.

DON'T OVERPLUCK; too-thin brows can make your face look too severe. Remember that most brunettes look best with a thicker brow than blondes. Naturally shaped brows, even when slightly asymmetrical, look subtly sexy.

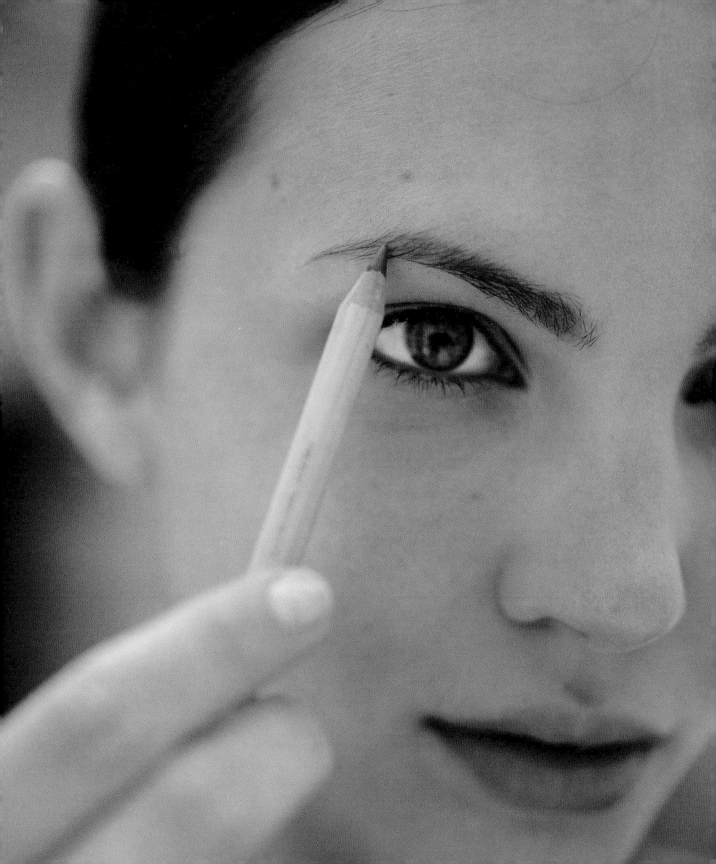

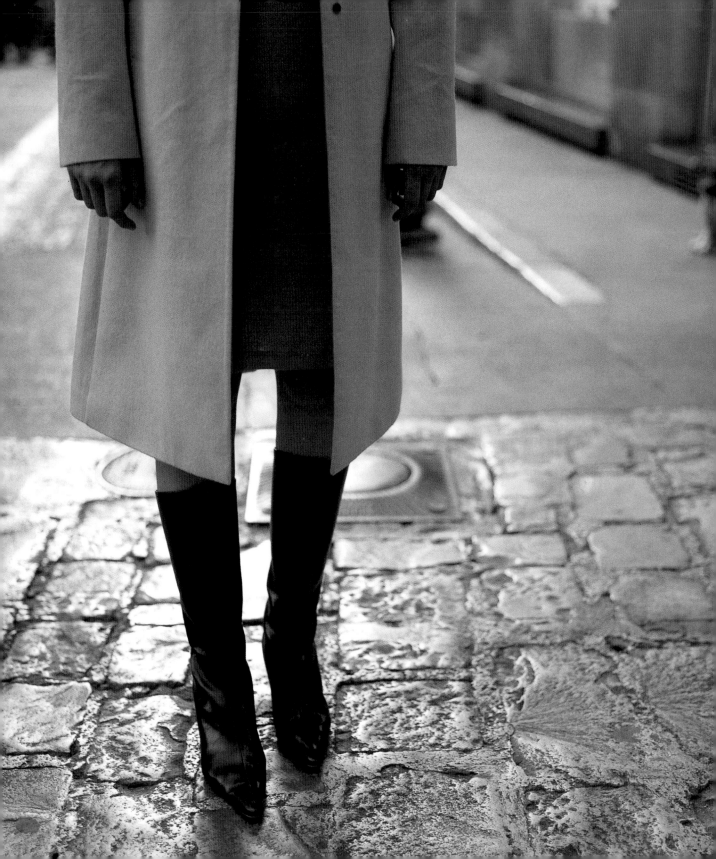

SIMPLIFY
YOUR WARDROBE: NEW YORK STYLE

I love New York. It's a jungle, but I love how I feel each morning when I wake up. Even in the dead of winter, it's my favorite city in the world. It sounds cliché to repeat it, but it's true: It has an energy like nowhere else. Though my schedule is insane, I thrive, like most New Yorkers, when I have too much to do.

I'll never forget my first day in Manhattan: I had come from Paris to open a salon on Madison Avenue for Jacques Dessange. I barely spoke English. It was about five o'clock when the cab left me off at Lexington Avenue and 81st Street in front of the apartment I was supposed to move into. I rang the bell, but of course no one answered, and there I was on the sidewalk, bewildered. I expected America to be like the movies: with huge iceboxes, big cars, four-lane freeways, Texas-sized ranches. Certainly nothing like cramped and funky Manhattan.

I went into the shop below to ask to use the phone. A beautiful woman, with long curly hair and big blue eyes, exclaimed, "I know you." It's impossible, I kept saying, I've just arrived from the airport, it's my *première visite*. But she insisted, "I know you. Your name is Frédéric. You cut my hair in Paris." It was October 8, 1983, the sun was setting on Lexington Avenue, the skyline lit a brilliant orange. I couldn't believe how good I felt. And that's when I knew that this was going to be my city.

New York at that time was stylish, yet very formal. Remember the eighties? Everyone was "done" to the ultimate degree. Nails were very long, very square. Hair was big and it never moved. Makeup, from lipstick to foundation, was matte—very aging, cakey, too obvious. And in fashion the trend was metallic fabrics that made people look very hard.

In this context, my taste, influenced by the easy life of Provence, was a breath of fresh air. I remember the first time Dawn Mello—former president of Bergdorf Goodman, one of New York's best specialty stores—walked

ADD A HEALTHY NEW VEGETABLE TO YOUR REPERTOIRE. TRY KALE, FENNEL, CELERY ROOT, OR BROCCOLI RABE.

REPLACE YOUR WATCHBAND. YOU'LL FEEL LIKE YOU HAVE A NEW WATCH FOR THE NEW YEAR.

LOOK OUT THE WINDOW FOR TEN SECONDS. DO THIS OFTEN DURING THE DAY TO REST YOUR EYES AND QUIET YOUR MIND.

TAKE A DAY OFF: SPEND IT WITH A NEW BOOK, A CASHMERE THROW, SOME HOT HERBAL TEA, AND A CRACKLING FIRE OR CANDLES

LOSE WINTER WEIGHT: FOR ONE WEEK, AS SOON AS YOU WAKE UP IN THE MORNING, DRINK A TALL GLASS OF WARM WATER WITH LEMON JUICE. THINK OF IT AS SPRING CLEANING FOR YOUR CELLS.

BUY A LIP BALM FOR EVERY HANDBAG OR COAT POCKET AND USE THEM RELIGIOUSLY.

EXERCISE FOR AT LEAST AN HOUR, NO MATTER HOW YOU'RE FEELING.

into the salon. She was used to having her hair set rather than simply blown out because she had been brainwashed into thinking that she had "difficult" hair. Too flat. Too heavy. Whatever. I changed all that. I showed her how to work her hair with her fingers. I took away her hairspray. And I freed her from the tyranny of tedious sessions under the hair dryer. This influential trendsetter who was one of the first to showcase Giorgio Armani's designs in this country had a tremendous influence on my career as well. Like Armani's unstructured suits, she sensed women would respond to my streamlined, natural approach to beauty. In 1989, she arranged for me to open my own salon at Bergdorf Goodman.

Today, the most stylish New York women I know have an understated, practical, easy elegance that captures the best qualities of French chic. It's not based on endless trips to the chicest boutiques—the most interesting women have the least time to shop. It's about editing.

Because of the diminutive size of apartments here, the New York woman doesn't have much closet space—she has no choice but be disciplined! But with a limited wardrobe each piece must work overtime, earning its keep by working for a range of occasions both casual and more formal. Cultivate a handful of tried-and-true outfits: a sleek pant suit under a big roomy coat, a smart sheath dress with sexy high boots, or a cashmere sweater with matching skirt and coat.

Ask yourself: Which are the three sweaters, three pairs of pants, and three skirts you love the most? Put them in the front of your closet. What are the three you wear least? Give them away (or at least put them away, in a box, out of sight). Get down to the essence of things.

One last thing: Get a lot of sleep. Particularly in cold weather, and particularly in a fast-paced town like Manhattan, it is the best thing you can do for yourself, period.

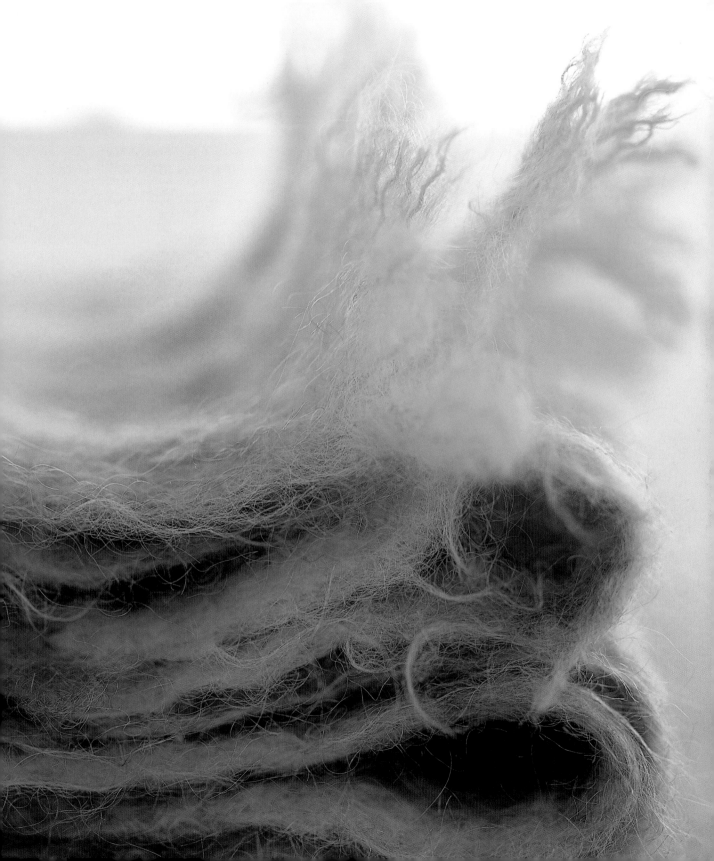

WINTER CHIC

Endless layers that must be piled on and peeled off are not modern. Adopt a look that works indoors and out. Here are some suggestions to weather wintry days in pared-down style.

* Have at least one classic cashmere or wool coat. Though understated, they're confident, powerful, and flattering. Whenever in doubt, think navy and black—you will never go wrong.

* Everyone needs a great raincoat with a detachable wool lining. You can throw it over everything, and it always looks chic. I prefer them in cement and loden green colors.

* A hat that you can crush in your bag and pull out when you need it is great. Pick one in microfiber that won't wrinkle.

* A great pashmina, wool, or cashmere scarf around your neck will keep you as warm as a huge puffy parka. Colors like pale peachy coral, bright deep blue, or garnet red can add the perfect unexpected flash of flattering color right around the face.

* Gloves in leather or suede, lined with cashmere or lambswool, are always elegant.

* Sturdy, wood-handled umbrellas with lots of coverage, preferably in black, cobalt blue, chocolate brown, or dark green. Logos on umbrellas are awful, like tacky wrapping paper on an otherwise elegant gift. They draw attention to themselves, not you.

* A fantastic roomy leather or wool handbag that you can throw over your shoulder, with enough room for your gloves and hat, is both stylish and practical.

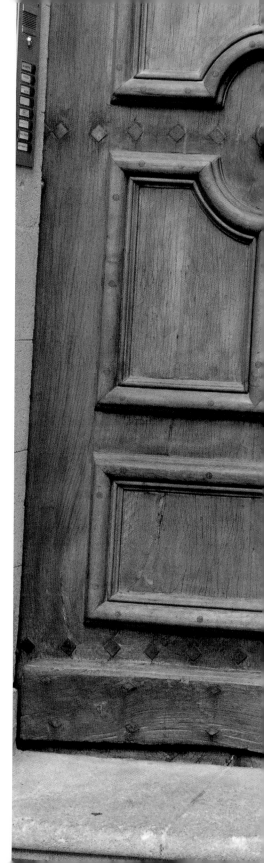

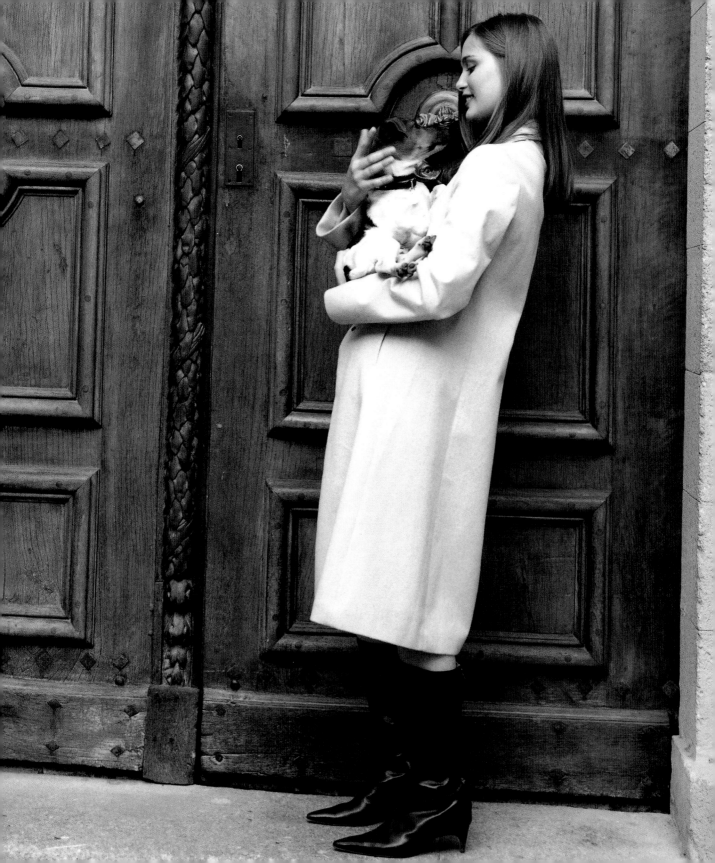

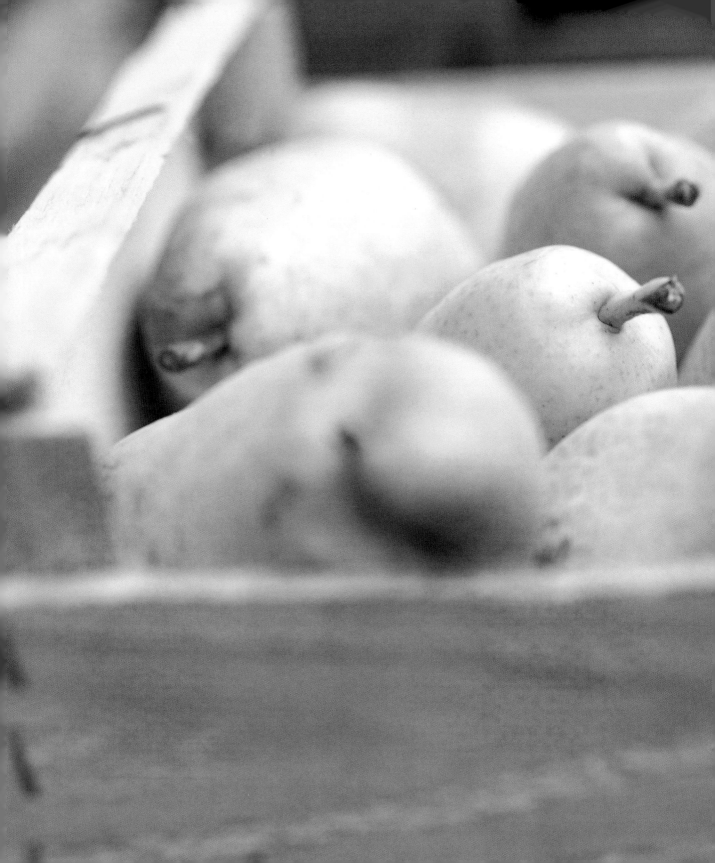

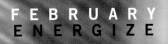

FEBRUARY
ENERGIZE

BUY A NEW FOUNDATION:
YOU MAY NEED A PALER
SHADE TO MATCH YOUR
WINTER COMPLEXION.

1

**GIVE YOURSELF A
CONDITIONING HAIR AND
SCALP TREATMENT,** OR HAVE
ONE AT YOUR SALON.

2

IF YOUR LIPS BECOME
CHAPPED, **USE A TOOTH-
BRUSH AND A LITTLE WATER
TO EXFOLIATE** THE DRY
SKIN, THEN SLICK ON SOME
LIP BALM.

3

In February, the pale winter light makes everything look more pristine and yet softer. At the same time, the mixture of crisp cold air and warm sunshine feels invigorating. Ah—this is the season to fall in love with life all over again. It's a surprising and uplifting sensation. No wonder Valentine's Day is in the middle of February!

Rediscover the energizing power of red and pink. The colors of passion, love, and romance will get you in a bright mood. Suddenly you'll want to wear a vibrant new sweater, carry a whimsical little handbag, or tie on a bright silk scarf—warm, yet fluid. Maybe it's also time to refresh—or rethink—your hairstyle with a fun new cut. And if you have let your exercise routine slide, take advantage of this unexpected boost of energy to jumpstart your fitness efforts.

Come on, the days are getting longer and you can't help but feel a rush of optimism.

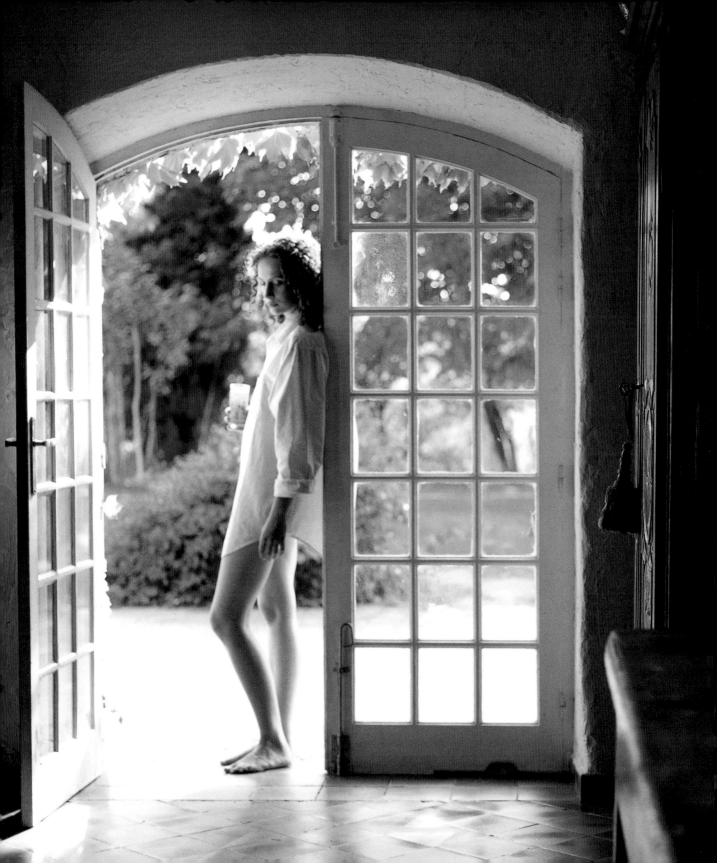

MAKE AN APPOINTMENT
FOR A VALENTINE'S DAY
MAKEOVER.

4

IF YOU CHANGE THE LENGTH
OF YOUR HAIR DRASTICALLY,
YOU MUST RECONSIDER ITS
COLOR AS WELL.

5

REMEMBER, THERE IS MORE
TO BE GAINED BY ELIMINATING
THAN BY ADDING.

6

GET
A GREAT CUT

Hair doesn't weigh that much. Yet get a good trim, and suddenly you feel a lot lighter. Younger, too, and more energized. The reason is simple: A great cut can give your hair instant oomph, vitality, and bounce. With each snip of the scissors, you sit up straighter, as if a load is being taken off your shoulders.

An overgrown mane feels heavy because it is out of balance. Hair lies flat in all the wrong places. It curls where it shouldn't. It falls forward when it should stay back. If you try to control it with gels, mousse, or hairspray, or if you try brushing it, blow-drying it in different directions, you are heading for a disaster. There is nothing worse than trying to fake shape and volume on hair that's simply outgrown and unruly. Your locks will never do what you want them to, they'll frizz or fall flat instead.

A good cut can make your hair swingy, bouncy, and full of life. It can make thin hair look thicker, and thick hair more manageable. It can make shiny hair look even shinier. It can enhance great hair color. Your face can look longer, or fuller, or more angular, as desired. You can erase or emphasize features. Your forehead, your nose, your cheekbones, or your jawline can become more or less prominent. In short, a good cut makes you more beautiful.

Volume placement is critical. For instance, if you have a long oval face, you should avoid cuts with too much fullness on top. (This is also true for men with receding hairlines.) In contrast, if you have a very round face, you'd look best with a bit of layering, to give an impression of volume and create a more balanced shape.

But hair cutting is not a matter of simple geometry. You can't choose the right shape for you by looking at a chart. Your hair is always in movement, and so are you. When I cut hair, I perform a little dance. I walk in circles around my client to observe her and her hair from every angle. I may ask her

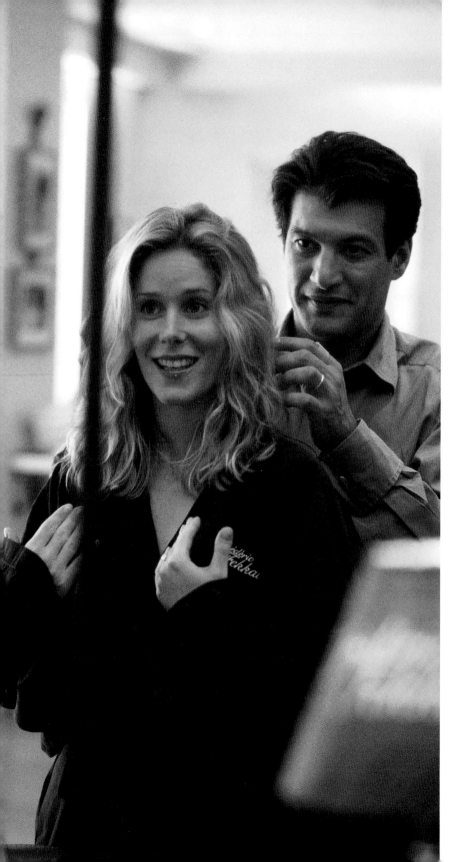

TIPPING SAVVY

The subject of tipping is one that makes many people very nervous. But tips do make up an important part of any stylist's salary, just as they do for waiters or taxi drivers. In general, tip between 15 and 20 percent of the total bill.

The main difference between the salon and a restaurant is that in the salon, you need to tip each person individually—15 to 20 percent needs to be divided among several people. I recommend calling the salon in advance to figure out exactly how much you'll be spending. Say your service costs $100, you'd tip the stylist $10, with $5 each for the stylist's assistant and the shampoo attendant.

Some salons have little envelopes at the front desk to put the tip in, as many people feel uncomfortable thrusting cash directly into the hands of their stylist.

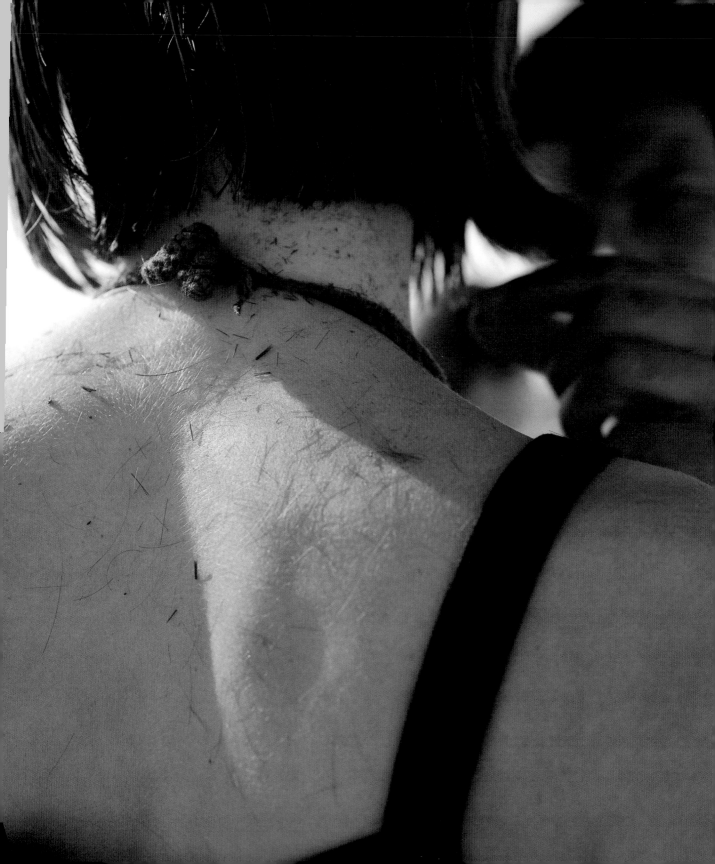

to stand up straight. Or sit back. Or walk about. I move with her. I bend forward and sideways. I make eye contact with her in the mirror. Then and only then can I determine what will work for her.

Ask yourself these questions to get the most from your haircut:

* **DO YOU HAVE GREAT BONE STRUCTURE?** You will look fabulous with short hair. Because short hair stands up straighter, it looks fuller, softening your handsome features as a result. Short layers play up this effect even further.

* **IS YOUR FACE SOMEWHAT NARROW?** Choose a midlength style, halfway between long and short. The longer your hair, the more layered it should be, to add volume at the sides.

* **DO YOU HAVE A ROUND FACE?** Favor longer hair to avoid looking chubby. A short cut can work if you keep the back longer than the front. If you are blessed with an angelic face and fine hair, short layers, cut at an angle on the sides, can look very sophisticated.

* **IS YOUR JAWLINE SQUARE?** Have your hair fall past your neck. The shorter your hair gets, the more pronounced your jawline. Never have bangs cut straight across; the squareness of full bangs will box in your face.

* **IS YOUR FACE HEART SHAPED?** You can carry off full bangs cut straight across the face. Long or short, it looks great, very Louise Brooks (the silent-film star).

* **IS YOUR NECK ON THE SHORT SIDE?** Your hair should never be too short in the back. Expose your neck indirectly, as you pull up your hair, with maybe a few tendrils hanging down. No matter how graceful your neck, an ultra-short cut in the back will make you look top-heavy.

LEFT: A BOB, CUT STRAIGHT ACROSS TO THE CHIN, IS A VERY STRONG, CHIC STYLE.

DRINK HOT HOMEMADE LEMONADE WITH HONEY IF YOU THINK YOU ARE GETTING A COLD. PAMPERING YOURSELF IS THE FIRST LINE OF DEFENSE AGAINST INFECTION.

7

THINK AHEAD. PLAN A SPECIAL VALENTINE'S DAY CELEBRATION NOW.

8

STAND WHILE YOU TALK ON THE PHONE. YOU'LL SOUND IN CHARGE AS WELL AS STRETCHING YOUR MUSCLES.

9

10 PLACE WOODEN TRAYS OR ZINC BUCKETS OF GREEN GRASS THROUGHOUT THE HOUSE.

11 HAND-WASH YOUR LINGERIE IN MILD SHAMPOO INSTEAD OF DETERGENT. IT'S LESS HARSH ON BOTH YOUR UNDIES AND YOUR HANDS.

12 TO FALL ASLEEP CONTENT, **READ POETRY BY RILKE, YEATS, OR RIMBAUD** BEFORE TURNING OFF THE LIGHT.

HAIRSTYLE BASICS

BANGS, NOT STRAIGHT ACROSS, but ones that fall to the side a bit, help balance out a long face. Really severe bangs are hard to pull off, and they cut the line of your face too harshly. But for most people, slightly wispy, angled bangs can be very sexy, and work to flatter the face.

LAYERS CAN GIVE VOLUME TO FINE HAIR, but you have to be very careful: In cutting layers, your stylist is cutting away hair, so it can end up too thin at the bottom. Blunter cuts mean more volume at the ends.

A BOB IS ALWAYS ELEGANT. It makes a statement, always looks pulled together, and can be so flattering. The straighter the hair, the better-looking the bob. Think of bobs at different lengths, depending on your face shape: chin-length or shoulder-length, for example.

SHORTER CUTS ARE MORE ENERGIZING and also sexier because you get a glimpse of the hairline, the ears, and the underside of the jawline. To men, a woman with short hair is very endearing. She gives the impression of being smart and adventurous, yet vulnerable.

SHORT, CHOPPY LAYERS LOOK FANTASTIC on almost anyone, emphasizing your bone structure, and making your eyes look larger and your lips fuller.

SHORT HAIR IS OFTEN EASIER to care for day-to-day, though you have to get it cut more often, about every four weeks.

IF YOU HAVE A LIFESTYLE THAT REQUIRES you to wash your hair frequently (athletes, for instance), short is for you.

RIGHT: SHORT LAYERS WITH A SOFT HAIRLINE GIVE A VERY SEXY, CONFIDENT, AND MODERN ATTITUDE.

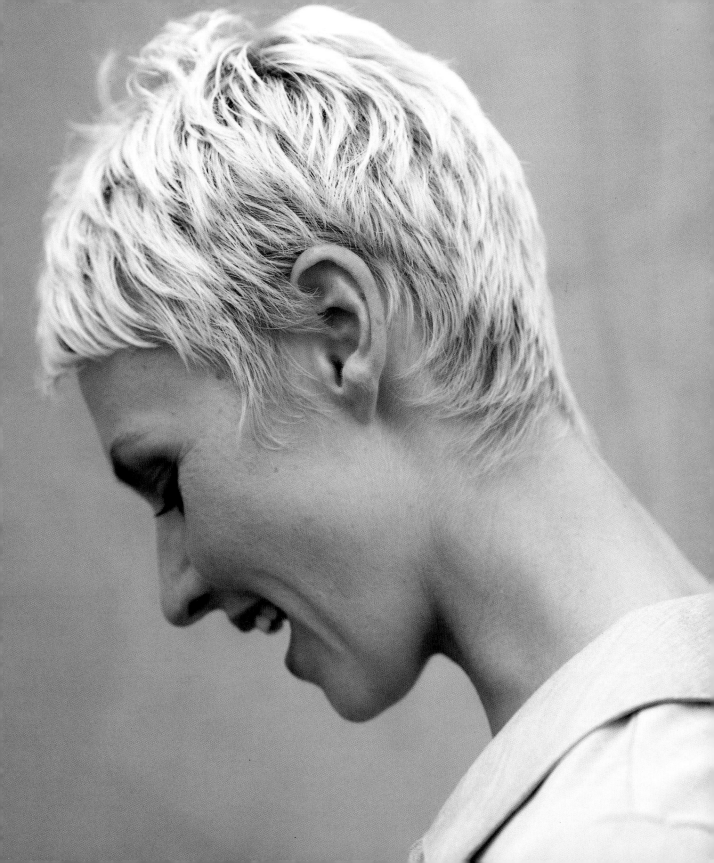

13   TAKE DANCE LESSONS.

14   GIFT IDEAS FOR VALENTINE'S
DAY: A PAIR OF FINE COTTON
PAJAMAS; AN ANTIQUE WATCH;
A SPA DAY; A MEANINGFUL
BOOK OR CD.

15   IF YOU EAT AT YOUR DESK,
**SEND E-MAILS RATHER THAN
MAKING PHONE CALLS.**
NOTHING'S WORSE THAN
TALKING WITH YOUR MOUTH
FULL—EVEN ON THE PHONE.

LONG HAIR CAN BE FLAT-OUT GORGEOUS. It's all in the shape of your face and in the cut you choose. As a rule, long hair that's all one length is chic and sophisticated. That said, long layers can also look fabulous, provided they're really long and blend in naturally to frame your face. Short layers look awful in long hair, the contrast is too great. If you get a trim every eight weeks or so, your long hair will stay healthy and bouncy.

For most women, cutting off their hair is fraught with anxiety. Many clients are desperately afraid of having their hair cut too short. In my experience, they're right to be scared. Many hairdressers do tend to cut hair too short. So it's very important to find a hairdresser with enough restraint to listen to you, and heed your wishes in terms of length.

On the other hand, be open if the topic of taking your style shorter comes up.

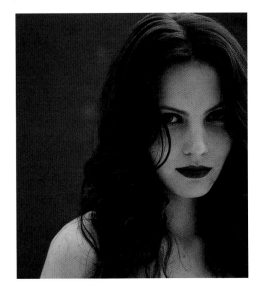

ABOVE: PROPERLY CUT, LONG LAYERS NATURALLY FRAME
THE FACE AND CAN BE VERY ALLURING. **RIGHT:** THE ANGLED
CUT OF THESE BANGS HELPS MAKE THIS ANGELIC ROUND FACE
LOOK MORE SOPHISTICATED AND SEXY.

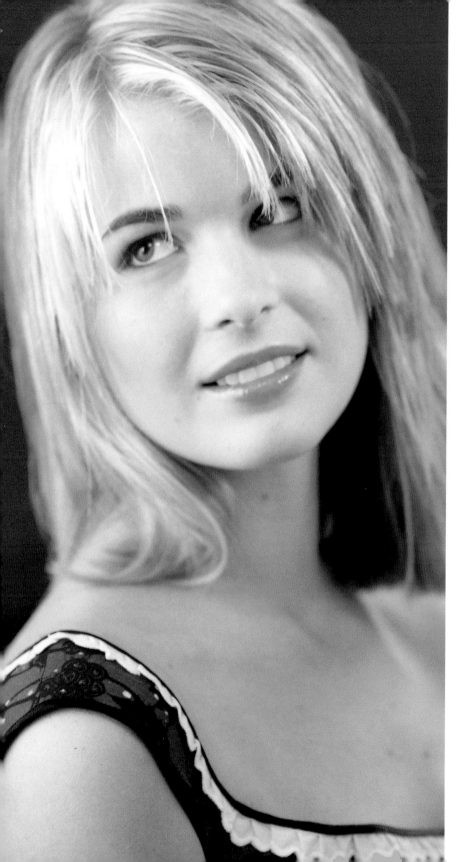

TRIMMING BANGS

Some of my most loyal clients don't come in when their bangs need a trim, despite the fact that it's a free service at our salon (this is probably the case at your salon, as well). The reason, simply, is time. So I teach people to do it themselves. The trick is to use a razor (the one you use to shave your legs is just fine) rather than scissors. The razor leaves a "piecey-er" line, which is much more forgiving and usually more flattering. If you must have blunt, blunt bangs, I'd go to the salon.

* WET YOUR BANGS with a spritzer or a wet brush.

* TAKE A LITTLE SECTION of bangs, and pull it down toward your nose, as far as it will go.

* TWIST IT just a tad.

* WITH THE RAZOR, cut it just below your eyes.

* THE WORST MISTAKE you can make is to cut your bangs too short, so always cut about an inch longer than the line you want—they will bounce up a bit. If it turns out to be too long, you can go back over it, but always err on the long side.

16

Unshined shoes
are the end of
civilization.

—DIANA VREELAND

17

ALTERNATE YOUR
CONDITIONER WITH A
RINSE THAT ELIMINATES
BUILD-UP.

18

TRY A WARM SOOTHING
HERBAL OIL FACIAL.

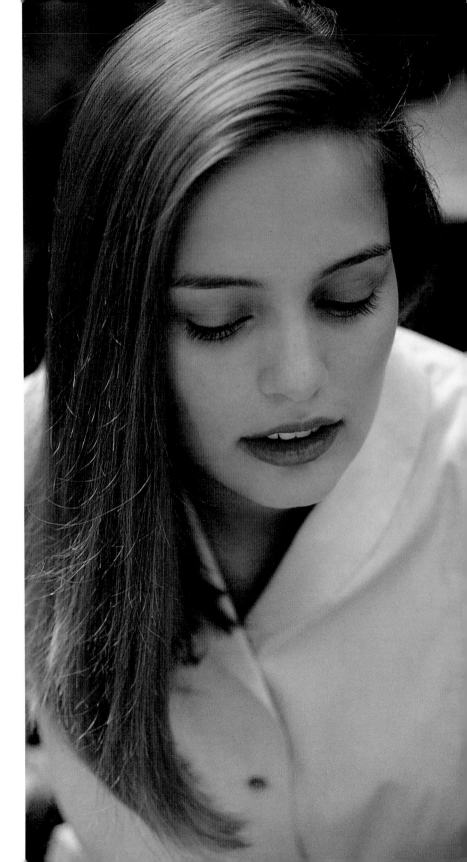

PARTS

* CHANGING THE DIRECTION OF A PART can completely change a woman's look. A part determines where the volume will occur in your hair. By moving a part, you can rebalance proportion to your advantage. If you need more volume at the top of your head (say you've got a very round face, for instance), and your hair normally parts in the middle, try parting it on the side. Now you've got a lot of hair going against its usual direction: The overdirection creates volume—right where you want it.

* YOU CAN DE-EMPHASIZE A WIDOW'S PEAK by redirecting the part.

* A MIDDLE PART WORKS with a lot of face shapes, except for a round one.

* A SIDE PART IS GREAT with most face shapes.

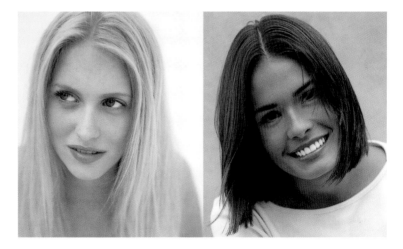

LEFT: A SIDE PART IS ALWAYS SOPHISTICATED.
ABOVE LEFT: A SLIGHTLY OFF-CENTER PART SOFTENS THE LOOK OF
SLEEK STRAIGHT HAIR. ABOVE RIGHT: THIS STYLE IS FUN AND
MODERN WITH A CENTER PART. IT CAN ALSO BE WORN
WITH A SIDE PART FOR A CLASSIC LOOK.

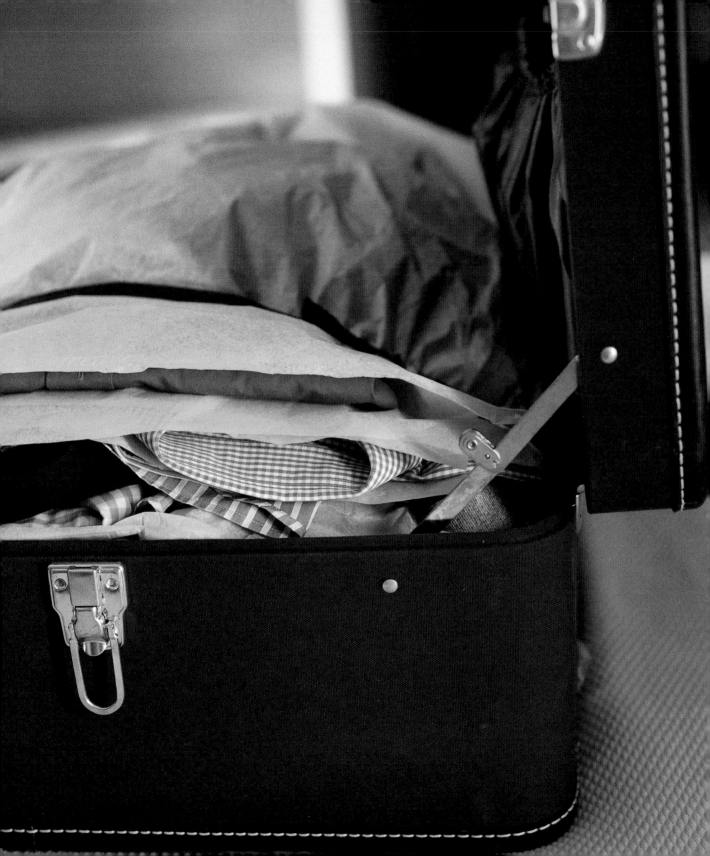

RE-ENERGIZE
THE WEEKEND GETAWAY

February can be unrelentingly gray. Growing up in France, we'd take a trip to North Africa, perhaps, or even Greece. Now a long weekend away completely renews me, a little sunshine (and a warm, slightly moist breeze) does wonders for the body and spirit.

Of course getting there in style can be more stressful than anything you put yourself through in the course of a workweek. A frazzled air traveler is never elegant. A great deal depends on how you pack, and how you dress for the trip. I always pack the night before; there's nothing more nerve-racking than scrambling around, trying to remember what to bring, knowing you have to make a plane. I travel so much that I've got it down to a science. I have traditional, somewhat heavier luggage. It makes for a less pleasant trip from the car to the check-in counter, but your things stay put inside them and, once you've arrived, they don't require ironing—which is no way to spend a vacation.

∗ **PACK MORE, NOT LESS**. It's so stressful to get somewhere and realize you're not prepared for a party, a business meeting, or an afternoon off, especially when you know the perfect item is at home, sitting in your closet. It's better to have a choice, despite the slightly heavier luggage.

∗ **A TRADITIONAL, HARD SUITCASE** is always better than a soft garment bag, which leaves clothes wrinkled and out of shape.

∗ **IF YOUR CLOTHES REALLY HAVE TO BE PERFECT**, fold them with tissue paper, in a hard suitcase.

∗ **BETWEEN GARMENTS**, throw in a couple of little lavender sachets, so everything smells fabulous when you arrive.

Gone are the days when we dress to travel, but do make an effort; just keep it simple, easy, elegant. For jet-setters of either sex, a pressed white

READY OR NOT?

To be ready for impromptu weekend escapes, always keep a waterproof toiletries bag packed with all your can't-live-without-it products. If you decide to take off on the spur of the moment—as you should—you will not waste precious time hunting around for your beauty essentials.

Must-haves include: toothpaste, sunscreen, moisturizer, shampoo (use it as soap, and even as fabric wash), conditioner (which, in a pinch, can double as finishing cream), cleanser, lipstick (a neutral shade that can be rubbed on cheeks as well), mascara, and a bit of perfume. Cotton swabs are also incredibly useful, multipurpose items; so are tweezers.

As for eyelash curlers and straightening irons, it all depends how high-maintenance you are.

**MAKE A SUMMERY DISH
FOR DINNER:** GRILLED FISH
SEASONED WITH BASIL,
COARSE SEA SALT, OLIVE OIL,
AND LEMON JUICE. GARNISH
WITH GREEN BEANS AND
BAKED TOMATO SLICES.

19

**COMPLIMENT FRIENDS WITH
A FEW SINCERE WORDS.**
NEVER ERR ON THE SIDE OF
BEING TOO EFFUSIVE.

20

FOR A TRIP TO THE TROPICS,
CONSIDER TAKING: *A NATURAL
HISTORY OF THE SENSES* BY
DIANE ACKERMAN; *THE
MAMBO KINGS PLAY SONGS
OF LOVE* BY OSCAR HIJUELOS;
*LOVE IN THE TIME OF
CHOLERA* BY GABRIEL GARCÍA
MÁRQUEZ; *ISLA NEGRA* BY
PABLO NERUDA (POEMS).

21

shirt, jeans, and black driving loafers, or a turtleneck and simple khakis are best, a perfect traveling wardrobe. You'll be comfortable, but you won't arrive looking or feeling disheveled. I must confess that when I travel overnight, I wear a Chinese silk suit that looks and feels like pajamas. It's lightweight, wrinkle-resistant, comfortable, and more important, chic!

* **AVOID HIGH HEELS,** and anything that really restricts your movement. A very structured jacket, for instance, or something very tight, is a poor choice.
* **MAKEUP AND HAIR SHOULD BE EASY, TOO.** Wear a ponytail, or use a barrette to tuck your hair out of the way.
* **WEAR PLENTY OF MOISTURIZER** and lip balm, and each time you go to the rest room, spritz a fine mist of mineral water over your face. Don't wear lipstick unless it's a neutral shade and very moisturizing.
* **EYE MAKEUP ISN'T GOOD ON AN AIRPLANE;** the dry air can make your eyes tear or itch, causing you to rub them, and you'll reach your destination looking as if you've been out all night.
* **TO LOOK WELL-RESTED,** rub on a little cream blush (not powder, it's too dry) just before you touch down.
* **A VERY LIGHT SCENT IS REFRESHING.** Anything heavy will bother other people. Never spray fragrance on a plane; bring a splash that you can dab on.

Give extra thought to your carry-on luggage. When you're making a short hop, you want something large enough to hold everything easily, with enough compartments to keep everything organized and easy to reach. A bag that's too big makes travel more difficult, and you don't want to be lugging a heavy load as you're rushing to make your connection. Classic leather tote bags hold up to the rough-and-tumble of airplane travel and always look great. Well-made nylon bags in black or navy (lighter colored nylon gets dirty and looks horrendous) work, too, and are more lightweight. Fabric bags are often too delicate and too easily soiled for serious traveling. Save them for the beach or a quick trip into town.

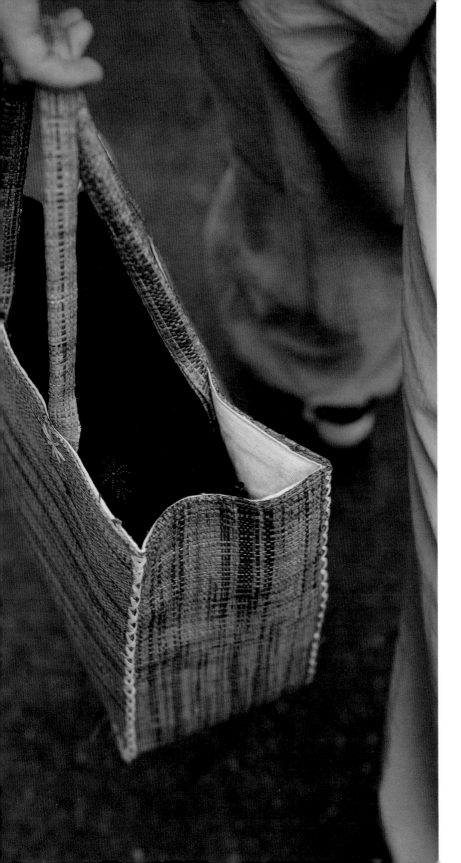

IN FLIGHT

Here is my list of what the well-stocked carry-on bag holds:

* Bottled water

* Cashmere: either a shawl or a sweater. Even in the heat of summer, airplanes can be freezing.

* A great book or favorite magazine

* A small spray bottle of citrus or lavender splash. Airplanes and airports can smell horrible.

* Toiletries bag with essentials

* Stationery, personalized if you have it, and address book. Flights are a wonderful time to catch up on correspondence.

* If you must take work along, don't pack more than you'll be able to finish. It will just weigh you down.

22 BRING YOUR OWN CD'S OR TAPES WHEN GETTING A MASSAGE. TRY ENNIO MORRICONE'S SOUNDTRACK FROM *THE MISSION*.

23 AFTER A SKI WEEKEND, **GET A HOT-STONE MASSAGE.**

24 **GO FOR A WALK IN THE SNOW** OR THE RAIN. DRESS WARMLY.

Take only the essentials in your carry-on. There's nothing worse than having to rummage around in the overhead compartment, trying to find something you need.

Even though it's February, don't let your pale winter complexion spoil your warm-weather weekend fantasy. Use a self-tanner, preferably the night before you leave. You'll arrive looking tanned and well-rested. It will affect how you feel, I promise. And why not trick yourself into thinking it's summertime by getting a pedicure in a fabulous coral-pink or fuchsia shade? You will begin to relax the minute the cab that's taking you to the airport pulls in front of your terminal.

SKI STYLE

I have warm, happy memories about skiing time: Wearing traditional mountaineer's gear. Enjoying the comfort and effortless style of snowboarding clothes. Admiring the technical perfection of skiing gear. But also, coming indoors in the moist air of a chalet after a day in the dry cold mountain air. Taking off my ski boots and putting on big slippers before settling down by the fireplace for a game of Scrabble. Eating tarte aux myrtilles in my blue flannel pajamas. Wrapping myself in a big cashmere blanket while the snow falls outside.

Today, skiers tend to go a little crazy with what they wear. Here are my recommendations:

IF YOU'RE GOING TO WEAR BRIGHT COLORS, stick with one or two, no more. Black is always classic for skiing.

GET HIP-LENGTH, extreme-ski coats that skim the body rather than hug it.

ALWAYS BUY COATS WITH LOTS OF POCKETS for sunscreen, lip balm, water, maybe even a cell phone.

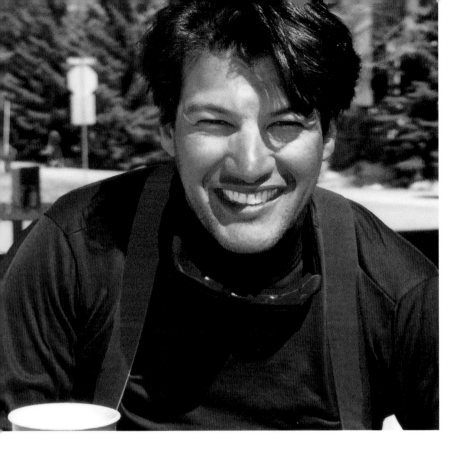

WHEREVER POSSIBLE, KEEP YOUR HAIR OFF YOUR FACE, neatly tucked into your hat. Ponytails always work.

SKI HATS CAN BE FUN, but try to stick to the two-bright-colors rule.

APRÈS-SKI, go for sport-styled clothes, maybe a bit closer to the body, in more muted colors: browns, blacks, grays, whites, loden green.

AT NIGHT, DO NOT WEAR MUCH MAKEUP—maybe a little blush or a touch of lip gloss, and very natural, casual hair.

The sun may be weaker in the winter, but when you're outdoors with snow all around you and at a high altitude, the sun can be quite strong. You need serious sunscreen to avoid sunburns and sun damage. Experiment with sport sunscreens to find one that suits your skin; for a sunny day of skiing, use at least SPF 30 in the most waterproof formula you can find, and reapply it often. Even cloudy days call for sunscreen. A lighter formula with an SPF 15 is ideal.

DO SOMETHING ARTISTIC TODAY. PAINT, WORK WITH CLAY, SKETCH, SNAP A FEW PICTURES, EMBROIDER . . . IT'S GOOD FOR THE SOUL.

25

Perfumes, colors and sounds echo one another.
—BAUDELAIRE

26

RE-READ A FAVORITE BOOK FROM CHILDHOOD.

27

PRACTICE BROTHERLY LOVE BY HOLDING THE ELEVATOR DOOR OPEN FOR LATE-COMERS.

28

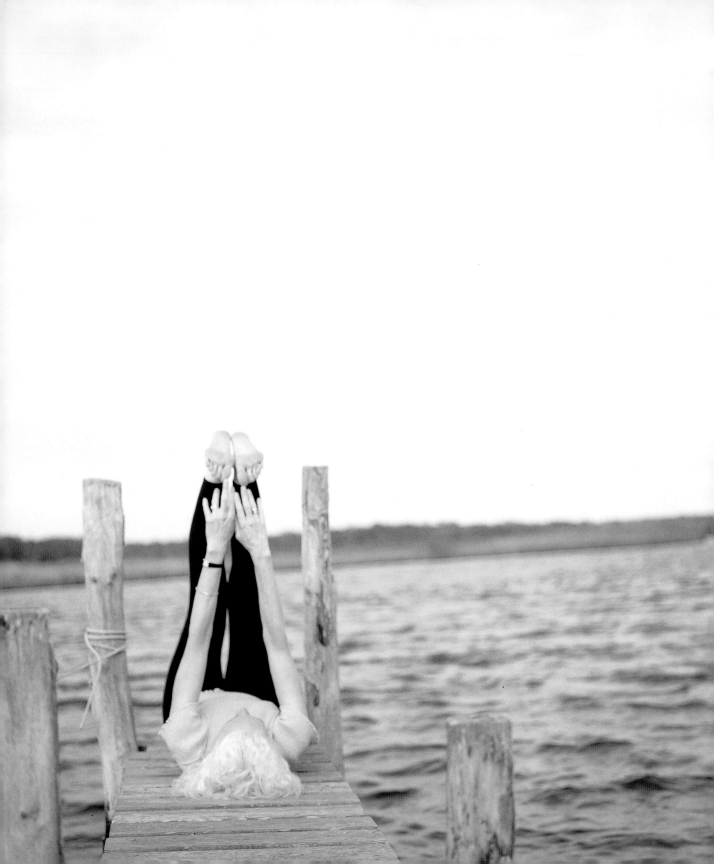

TAKE A FITNESS BREAK

By the middle of February, almost everyone I know could use a little more discipline in the exercise department: When the weather's not so great, it's easy to ignore your body, to spend that extra hour at your desk rather than at the gym or yoga studio. So even a short weekend away in the sun is the time to re-awaken that side of yourself. Take advantage of the warm weather to do yoga outside, first thing in the morning. Take a walk on the beach. Get a massage. Eat well: fruit, vegetables, whole grains, fresh things. The exercise part, especially, might feel like work at first, but it's well worth it.

February is a great time to test a new fitness routine. Mix up your cardiovascular workout with weight-training, or try something new. If you haven't tried the Pilates method, maybe now is the time. This form of exercise focuses on lengthening rather than just strengthening your muscles. Developed by a dancer, Pilates is based on a series of machines that use traction and pulleys, though some trainers prefer you work with your own body to provide the resistance necessary. Either way, an hour-long routine will help you adjust your posture and carry yourself in a whole new way.

Yoga is another exercise that's both relaxing and invigorating. Master the slow yet deliberate moves of this traditional Indian workout and your body is sure to become more flexible, and your mind less restless. And if you're used to a more rigorous workout, find a yoga instructor who balances meditation and breathing with stretching and aerobic movement.

The most efficient way to get an energy boost and enjoy some relaxation is reflexology, a form of acupuncture that originated in China, though no needles are involved. It is based on the theory that pressure points for all the major organs and body parts are found in the feet. As the therapist massages your soles, he is stimulating different parts of your body.

RIGHT: I LOVE TO EXERCISE OUTSIDE, ESPECIALLY FIRST THING IN THE MORNING.

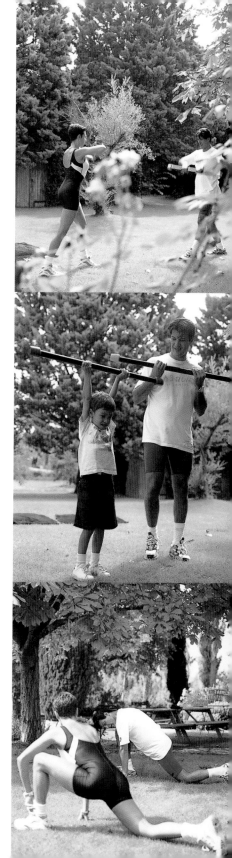

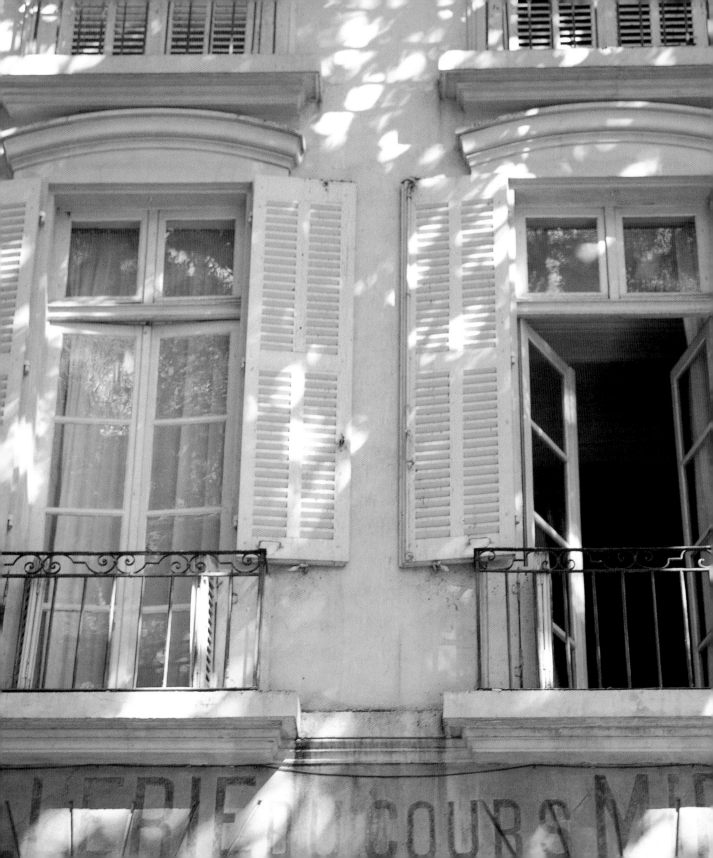

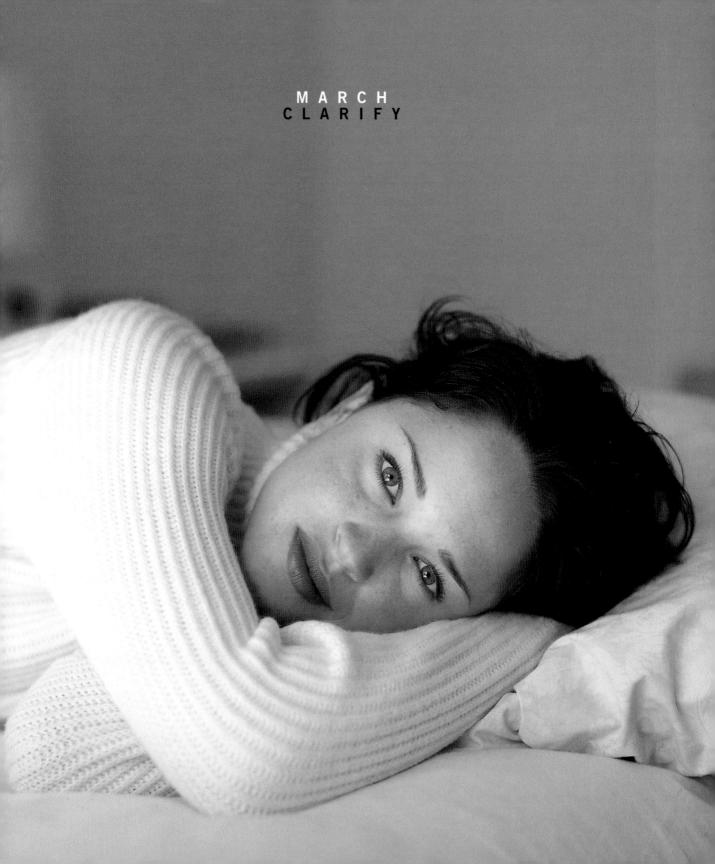

MARCH
CLARIFY

1   **HAVE A SALON BLOWOUT** FOR NO SPECIAL REASON OTHER THAN TO FEEL PAMPERED.

2   **SORT THROUGH YOUR LIPSTICKS** AND THROW OUT ANY YOU HAVEN'T USED IN TWO MONTHS.

3   **MAKE A LIST** OF THE OSCAR-NOMINATED FILMS YOU WANT TO SEE BEFORE THE BIG NIGHT.

March is a transitional month. We're all waiting for the last lingering days of winter to finish and eagerly anticipating the beginning of spring. Now is the time to clarify your look and re-create yourself. By the time April rolls around, you'll be ready to stride into spring with energy and a clear outlook.

What worked for you this winter—and what didn't? Are your clothes sending the message you want them to? If not, clarify that message by paring away vestiges of an old or outdated look. Re-evaluate your wardrobe of accessories. One or two fantastic additions like a brightly colored barrette in a wonderful snakeskin or a passe-partout handbag in a clever combination of materials like satin and straw can make a stronger statement about who you are than a dresser full of nondescript accessories. Keep this in mind as you consider what you'll be adding to your closet for the new season.

RIGHT: FOCUS YOUR LOOK ON STRONG, SIMPLE PIECES AND EVERYTHING WILL FALL IN PLACE.

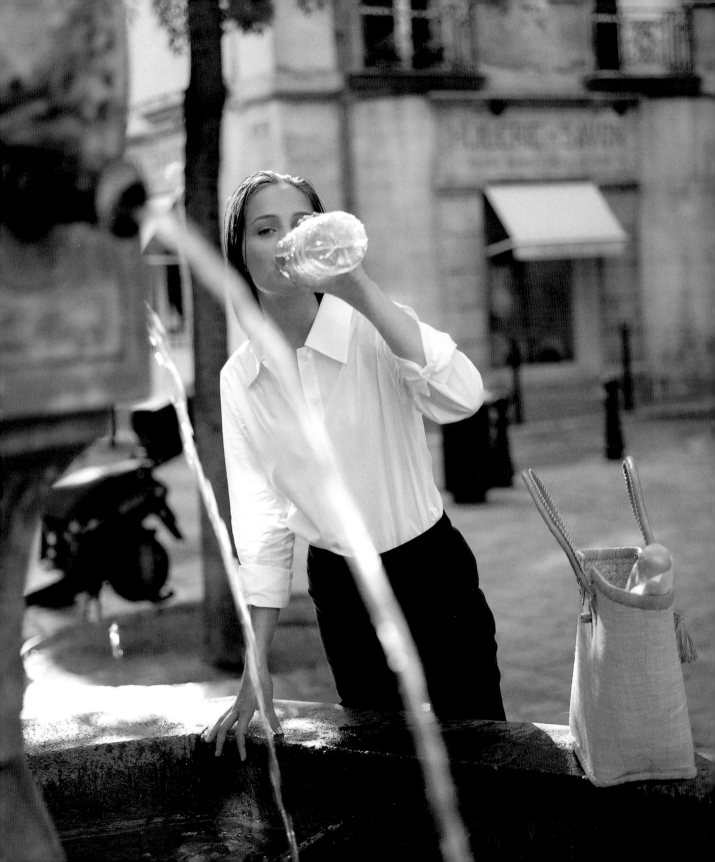

APPLY A HAIR MASK AND KEEP IT ON AS LONG AS POSSIBLE. THE DRIER YOUR HAIR IS, THE LONGER YOU SHOULD LEAVE IT ON, AND THE SHINIER, HEALTHIER, AND BOUNCIER YOUR HAIR WILL BE.

4

BE SELFISH. ONCE A DAY, DO AT LEAST ONE THING JUST FOR YOU.

5

BE GENEROUS. ONCE A DAY, DO AT LEAST ONE THING FOR SOMEONE WHO NEEDS HELP.

6

This could be the time to clarify your hair color as well. If you've been getting highlights for a long time you may have moved very far away from the look you originally sought; sometimes going back to ground zero (or what you remember as ground zero) and building on that tone with high- or low-lights is the way to go. There's certainly no better way to shake off the winter doldrums than with a shining, lustrous, richly colored head of hair. In fact, a great new hair color might just be the ultimate accessory!

In March, willy-nilly, we all focus on Los Angeles for what has become the most-hyped, most-loved worldwide event: the Oscars. It's the biggest glamour-fest of the year. And just in time, too. As winter drags on, a taste of glitter is just what the doctor ordered. But more important, we watch the stars for hints of their personalities beneath the diamonds and designer gowns. Who has the confidence to allow her beauty to shine? Who seems lost inside a too-grand dress or too-fixed hairstyle? When I work with women before the Oscars I often urge them to do less—take off one item of jewelry, stay away from elaborate coiffures. To me, the most glamorous women are those who wear their finery with the same casual chic they radiate in a pair of jeans. It's a matter of having confidence in yourself, your look, your style as *you* have defined it.

CASUAL CHIC

Though I am based in New York, my second flagship salon is in the center of the entertainment industry's wellspring of glamour—Beverly Hills. The more time I spend there, the more appreciation I have for the unique sense of confidence and style that seems like second nature to so many of the clients I see there.

I always point to the effortless chic of well-dressed, put-together French women as my models, but the women in California may be their American equivalents.

Contrary to popular belief, glamour in Los Angeles is easygoing. Everything

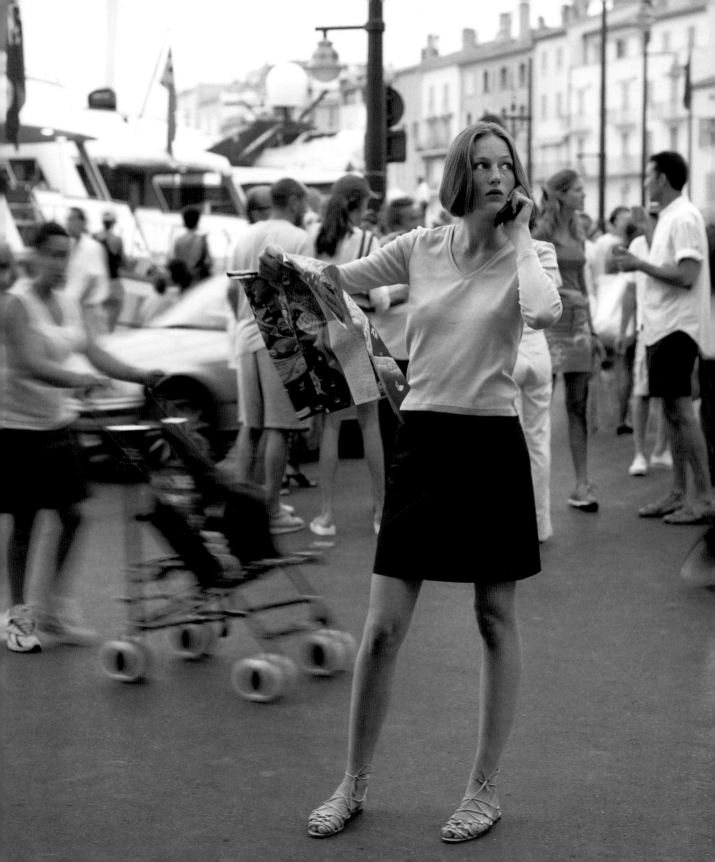

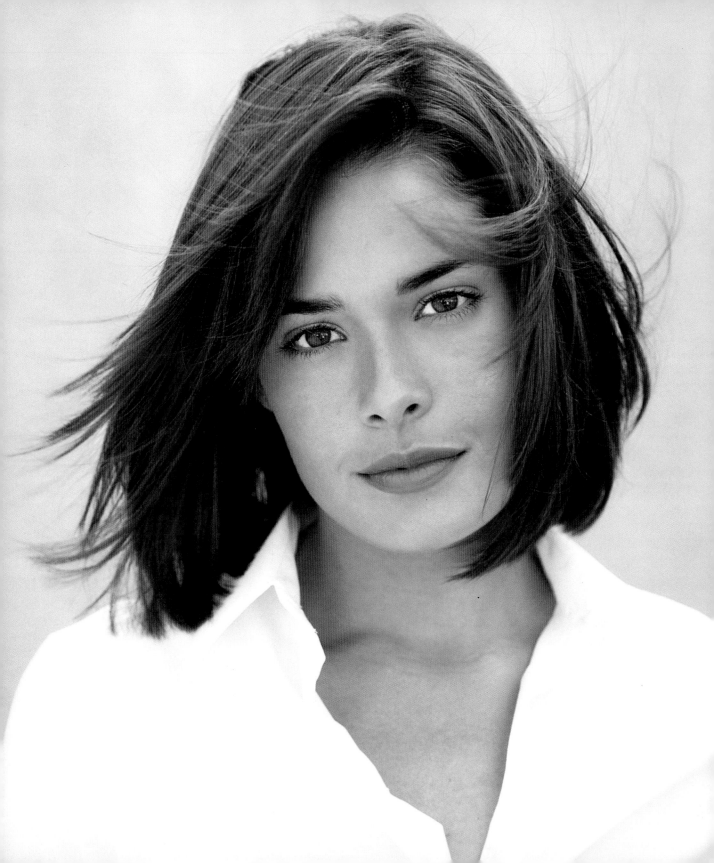

is a little more carefree. No wonder: Drive west on any boulevard, and you end up at the beach. Along the way, you can hear the wind blowing, the birds singing, the leaves rustlng. On the whole, life seems less stressful. People seem less worried. Blonder, too, and with longer hair and subtly enhanced features. Heavy makeup and showy jewelry are old Hollywood; today, Beverly Hills is home to some of the most natural and unpretentious people I know.

A sense of glamour and ease, though, doesn't exclude making some effort. Celebrities, who are constantly photographed, scrutinized, and envied, are well aware of the importance of looking polished, even at their most casual. For evening, or for big events, they affect a look that's elegant, but sort of bare—that doesn't try too hard. Glamour, California-style, boils down to three indispensable elements: sexy, glossy, casually styled hair with movement; a toned, fit body; and a deliberately underdone approach to makeup and clothes. It's youthful, easy, and confident.

GREAT HAIR COLOR
NO MATTER WHO YOU ARE

March is also the perfect time for giving your hair a color boost. As the light starts to change with the coming of spring, many of my clients are tempted to rethink their hair color. Many want to go lighter to match the new, paler colors they're buying for their spring wardrobes, or simply want to look brighter, lighter, in anticipation of the season.

But lighter isn't always the right direction. Hair color is as much about dark as it is about light; it's the interplay of those two elements (like the dappled sunlight under the *platane* trees in Provence) that makes your hair look alive, healthy, and well kept—it's not about applying a flat mask of color. Hair with depth, which you can get only from the contrast of dark and light, is natural, glamorous, and above all, sexy. Whether you have your color done in a salon or do it yourself at home, the goal should be marrying your natural hair

Always leave them laughing when you say good-bye.
—GEORGE M. COHAN

7

BUY FOUR BUNCHES OF YOUR FAVORITE FLOWERS AND MAKE A BIG BOUQUET FOR YOUR DINING ROOM TABLE.

8

GIVE YOURSELF A HOME FACIAL BY HOLDING YOUR FACE OVER A LARGE BOWL CONTAINING HOT CHAMOMILE TEA. STEAM FOR FIVE MINUTES. PAT YOUR FACE DRY. LET IT COOL BEFORE APPLYING MOISTURIZING CREAM.

9

10

IF YOU ARE THINKING OF A NEW HAIRSTYLE, **START PULLING PICTURES FROM MAGAZINES.**

11

PUT LAVENDER SACHETS UNDER YOUR PILLOWS DURING THE DAY. YOU'LL SLEEP BETTER, AND EVERYTHING WILL SMELL CLEAN, FRESH, AND SUMMERY.

12

IF IT HAS BEEN MORE THAN SIX WEEKS, **HAVE YOUR BROWS PROFESSIONALLY SHAPED.**

color with dye or bleach (or both) to achieve contrast. With clients whose hair is either too bleached or too dyed, a lot of what we do involves heightening contrast.

Hair should never look flat or over-colored and it also needs to be appropriate to your skin tone. You couldn't imagine Sophia Loren as a blonde, could you? Even if you were blond as a child, you shouldn't necessarily be blond as an adult: In all likelihood, your skin tone has changed along with your natural hair color. The downside to a major color change is maintenance, unattractive roots, fading, generally less-healthy hair. And there's nothing worse than hair that's been bleached, stripped, and colored again; it gets porous and plastic-looking. A good colorist takes things slowly, erring on the side of too little color. Just as with a great hairstylist, the best way to find a great colorist is to ask someone with incredible hair color where they had it done.

* **COLOR SHOULD NEVER BE OPAQUE**, because it never is in nature. You want to achieve as much transparency, as many layers of color, and as many different shades as possible.

* **YOU GROW OUT COLOR JUST LIKE YOU GROW OUT A HAIRCUT**, it takes some time, and a little extra thought.

* **NEVER COLOR YOUR ENTIRE HEAD OF HAIR JUST TO DO IT.** Virgin hair is always incredible; you can't do better than your own shine. Always keep some of your virgin hair.

GOING BLOND

Women think that blondes have more fun. Oh yes? Before you go blond, think how much fun it's going to be to sit in the colorist's chair for hours every four weeks. That said, blond can be very beautiful. If you're ready to make the commitment, then take the plunge, bearing in mind:

RIGHT: THESE BLOND HIGHLIGHTS SHINE BECAUSE OF THE VIRGIN HAIR ON THE BACKGROUND.

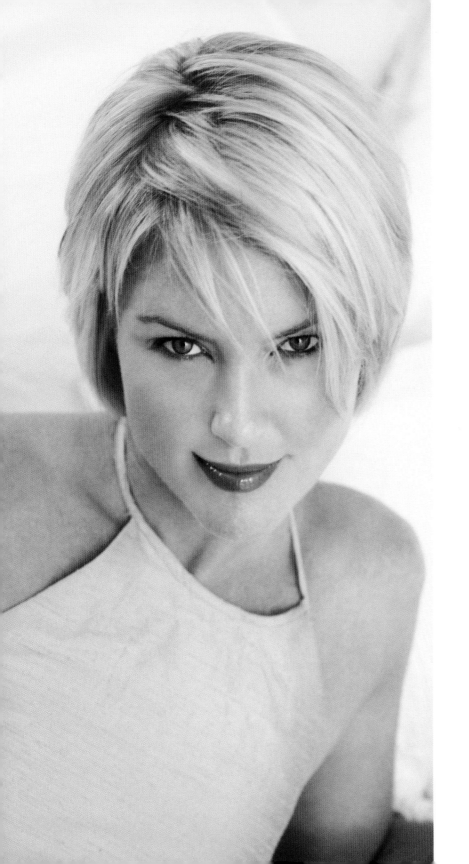

PROTECTING HAIR COLOR

Once you've spent precious time and hard-earned money getting your hair color right, protect it between applications. Always use gentle shampoos and conditioners designed specifically for colored, chemically treated hair.

* IF YOU ARE IN THE SUN, wear a hat. There are also good color-protection sprays that are sprayed onto wet or dry hair.

* SWIMMING in a chlorinated pool can turn your hair color into something practically unrecognizable. Protect it by applying a conditioning mask all over your hair before you swim. Or do as they do in Provence, use olive oil.

* RINSE YOUR HAIR thoroughly in cold water, after going in chlorinated water.

* SWEAT AND SALT WATER can also affect hair color: Special rinses, when used in conjunction with cold water, can get rid of any residue.

* COLOR-ENHANCING shampoos and conditioners can maintain your color and make it last longer.

AT-HOME COLOR

Color out of the box is not a bad idea, as long as you don't take big risks. Stick with something close to your natural shade and it's hard to go wrong. Follow the instructions to the letter. What would possess someone to do otherwise is beyond me, but people do, and we see the disastrous results in the salon.

* **SEMI-PERMANENT COLORS** are much more forgiving than the permanent ones, as they wash away over time, making the roots less noticeable.

* **WE ALL LOVE THE IDEA of** natural vegetable dyes, but they tend to be drying, and the color can take three hours to set.

* **HENNA LOOKS GREAT ON SOME PEOPLE**, but not on everyone. It's also practically impossible to get rid of the color, once you've applied it. Be prepared to let it grow out or cut your hair short, if you decide to change your color again.

* **IN GENERAL**, the color should be a little brighter around the face, more subtle in the back.

* **TOO MUCH BLEACH** makes blondes look ashy. It's bad for most skin tones.

* **BEWARE OF WHAT I CALL "PARK AVENUE HIGHLIGHTS"**: white bleach-blond streaks. They wash out your skin tone like nothing else. Instead try honey blond, buttery blond, even champagne blond. (White bleach-blond highlights look natural only on women who are still natural blondes.)

* **THE DOUBLE PROCESS** necessary to lighten hair and create highlights within that new color is hard on your hair, but unfortunately, the single process isn't always enough to get a natural blond look.

* **ON GRAY HAIR**, a single process works beautifully, because the white hairs stand out and work as highlights.

* **IF THE BLOND IS TOO OVERDONE**, reverse the process slowly by growing out the roots and adding darker low-lights.

GOING DARKER

Recently I've found more and more clients becoming receptive to a suggestion of deep, rich, dramatic color. Dark hair looks best with lots of contrast, with many different tones in it. When hints of color reflect off one another, the darkness acquires depth and vibrancy. Dark hair is pretty with pale skin. Think of women like Isabelle Adjani, Courteney Cox Arquette, Andie MacDowell. But dark hair also looks great with dark skin, particularly when highlighted with discreet brown sugar, honey, or tobacco streaks.

Keep the following in mind:

* **TO GIVE DARK HAIR DIMENSION**, opt for "low-lights," rather than highlights. These darker strands shape and personalize hair.

RIGHT: RICH BROWNS LOOK FANTASTIC AGAINST PALE SKIN AS WELL AS TAWNY COMPLEXIONS.

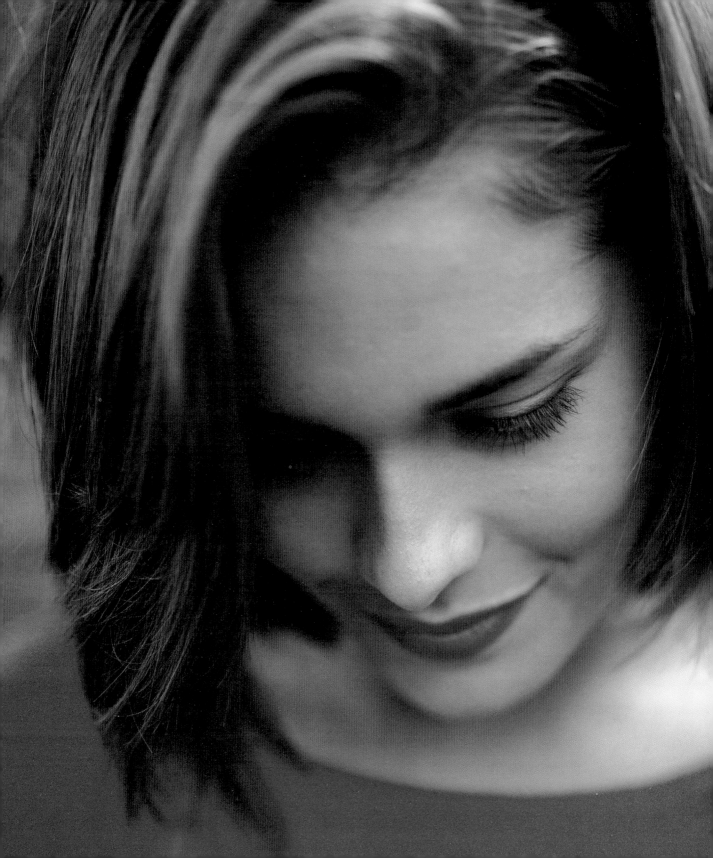

13 INSTEAD OF READING THE NEWSPAPERS OVER BREAK-FAST, **READ A FEW PAGES OF A BOOK YOU LOVE** AND CATCH UP WITH THE NEWS LATER ON THE INTERNET.

14 **BAD HAIR DAY?** WEAR A SATIN, LEATHER, OR VELVET BARRETTE IN YOUR HAIR.

15 **PERFECT A SIGNATURE DISH,** PREPARING IT OVER AND OVER, EVERY TIME YOU ENTERTAIN. ONCE YOU CAN DO IT WITH YOUR EYES CLOSED, TAKE ON A NEW ONE.

* **HIGHLIGHTS AT JUST THE ENDS OF DARK HAIR** are also flattering, as if you've been in the sun.
* **REMEMBER THAT HIGHLIGHTS**, no matter how dark your color, can get to be too much, both visually and for the health of your hair. You never want to lose the natural luster and shine of your hair.
* **HAIR THAT'S DYED TOO DARK** is incredibly difficult to fix. You have to grow out the roots patiently.

GOING RED

Worldwide, red is the most popular choice in haircoloring, as well as the most available and the easiest to accomplish. It is also a little more forgiving than blond, in terms of maintenance and roots. For these reasons, it's not always as unique as you might think. It's also not flattering on everyone.

* **FAIR SKIN** is lovely with red, particularly coppery, strawberry shades.
* **DARK SKIN TONES** look best with mahogany red or auburn shades.
* **VERY ARTIFICIAL,** wine reds are rarely flattering, and much too common.
* **IF A RED'S TOO RED,** highlights can make it more coppery, or more strawberry blond.
* **RED CAN BECOME OXIDIZED** and get too brassy or too pink. Toners bring it back. Most toners take only about five or ten minutes to work, and are almost as easy to use as shampoos.
* **IF YOU HAVE AN OLIVE COMPLEXION**, or lots of yellow undertones in your skin, don't go red.

RIGHT: IF YOU DECIDE TO GO RED, TAKE YOUR CUES FROM NATURAL REDHEADS.

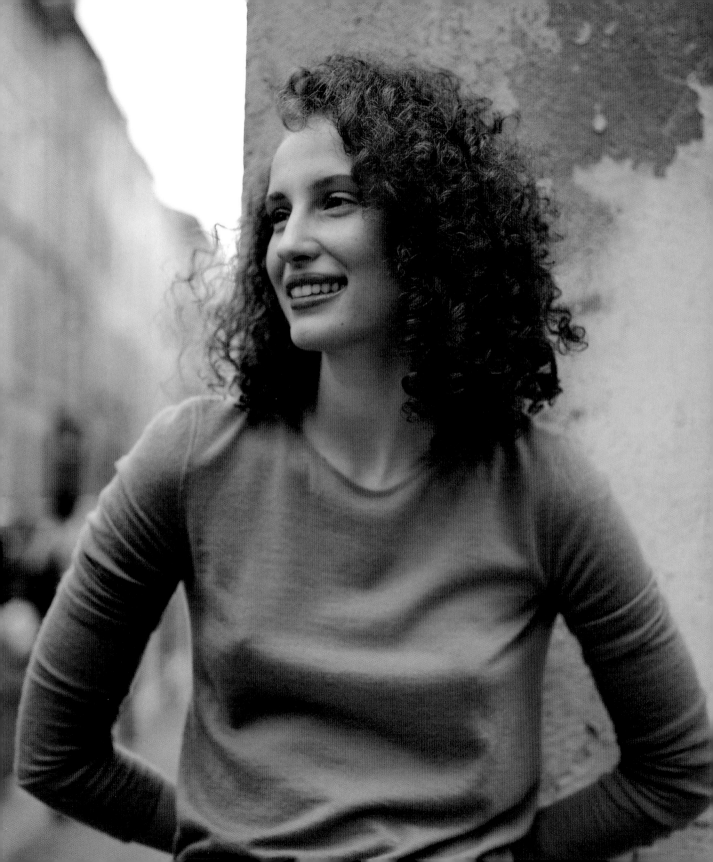

16 BUY A NEW SET OF MAKEUP BRUSHES.

17 FOR INSTANT STYLE, **COMBINE A CLASSIC BOTTOM WITH A MORE FASHIONABLE TOP.** THE OTHER WAY AROUND IS MORE TRICKY TO PULL OFF.

18 GREAT MUSIC TO DRIVE TO: FRANK SINATRA, AARON NEVILLE, TONY BENNETT, THE THREE TENORS, SERGE GAINSBOURG, MILES DAVIS, ARETHA FRANKLIN, BONNIE RAITT, SHERYL CROW, BILLIE HOLIDAY.

THE CASE FOR GRAY HAIR

If you've got just a few gray hairs, don't go for overall permanent color. Instead, opt for low-lights or highlights. Fifty to sixty percent less gray will make you feel younger while still looking natural, and you won't have to go to a salon nearly so often.

* **DON'T USE PERMANENT COLOR** until you are at least 30 percent gray.
* **IF AT LEAST 50 PERCENT OF YOUR HAIR IS GRAY**, it might be time to go with the flow and embrace gray. Take a good long look; more often than not, gray is chic and flattering.
* **IF YOU DO DECIDE TO STAY WITH YOUR NATURAL GRAY**, maintain it well. Rinse with apple cider, which prevents gray hair from yellowing.
* **A SPECIAL BLUE SHAMPOO** used once a month can leave gray hair brighter and more shiny.

Emma Thompson came to see me when she was growing out her hair color with the idea to phase it out altogether. Her hair was almost completely gray, which is the right time to go natural, but she needed to find a new style to keep her looking sexy and chic. She specifically asked for something unconstructed, easy, and versatile, with lots of movement. I cut her hair along the lower edge of her neck, angling the bangs shorter at the brow, going longer toward the cheekbones, all the way down to the neckline. We did some shorter layers near the crown, angling down toward the hairline—a modern shag. When it was done, she ran her fingers through her hair and flashed a broad smile. Her eyes shining, she turned around and gave me an enormous hug. That's what's great about cutting hair: You can make someone feel very special—even a movie star.

RIGHT: COMBINE A MODERN HAIRCUT WITH GRAY HAIR AND THE RESULT IS AMAZING!

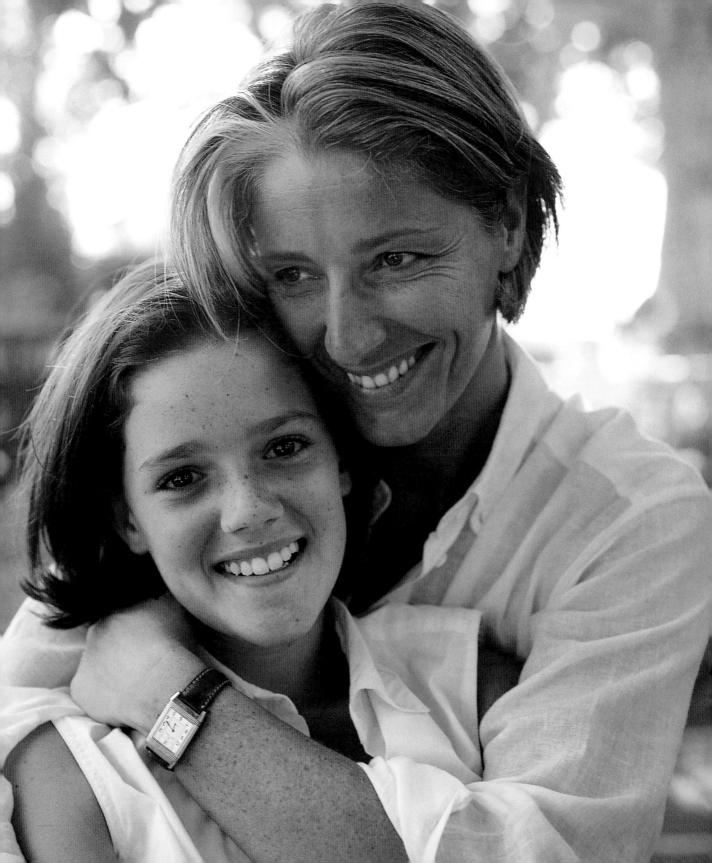

19

20

REMEMBER THAT TALKING ON A CELL PHONE DOESN'T MAKE YOU LOOK IMPORTANT. THE PRESIDENT OF THE UNITED STATES DOESN'T CARRY ONE.

21

TO CELEBRATE THE OFFICIAL END OF WINTER, **GIVE YOUR BODY A FRIENDLY WAKE-UP CALL:** TAKE A SHOWER THAT'S SLIGHTLY COLDER THAN USUAL, THEN DRY YOURSELF IN A WARM FLUFFY TOWEL.

THE CONFIDENT FACE

With clarity comes confidence, and a look that is more polished than "made up." It is, however, a stronger look than the very natural face on page 26.

This chic face brings attention to the eyes and mouth, letting the cheeks and face act as a backdrop for glamorous appeal. Usually you want to focus on one particular feature, not the eyes and the mouth at the same time. The reason this face works so well, even though it betrays that rule, is because the lip and eye colors are monochromatic, that is, the same color. You can even use a strong polish on your hands if it matches the color on the eyes and lips. When you're choosing the colors for this look, keep this monochromatic idea in mind and try to pick tones that match each other as closely as possible.

EYES Pick a rich shadow like a bronze, navy, or clove, and apply it across the entire eyelid. Sweep a thin line under the eye as well. Blend well.

CHEEKS Leave your cheeks bare, excepting what you would normally use (like concealer) to even out the skin tone.

LIPS Match your lipstick color with your eye shadow. Apply the lipstick evenly so that the color is smooth across the lip (do not use any gloss).

NAILS Again, pick a color that matches your lipstick and eye shadow as much as possible. You can use the same color on the fingers and toes.

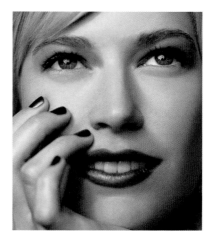

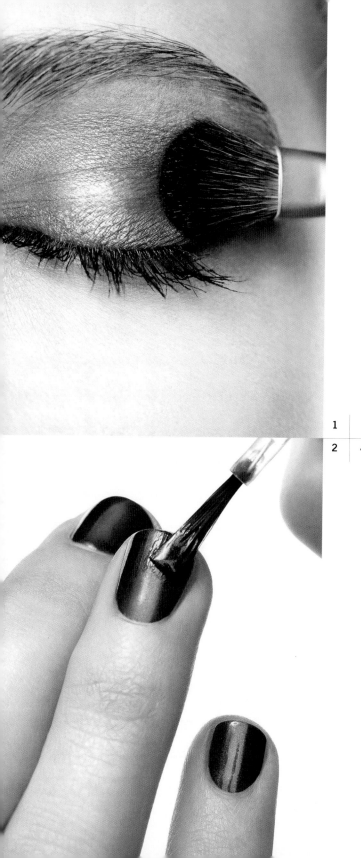
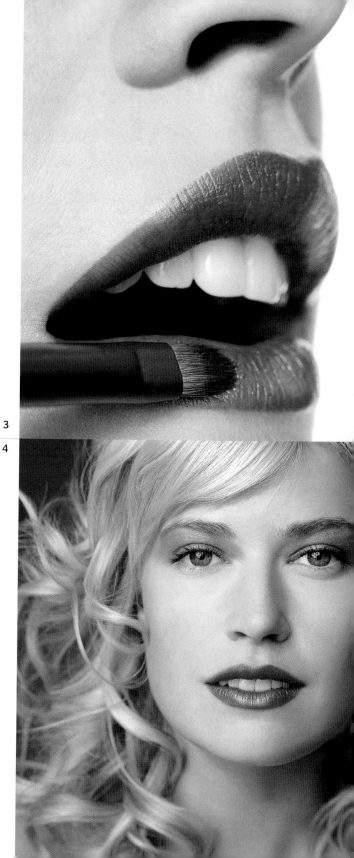

1 | 3
2 | 4

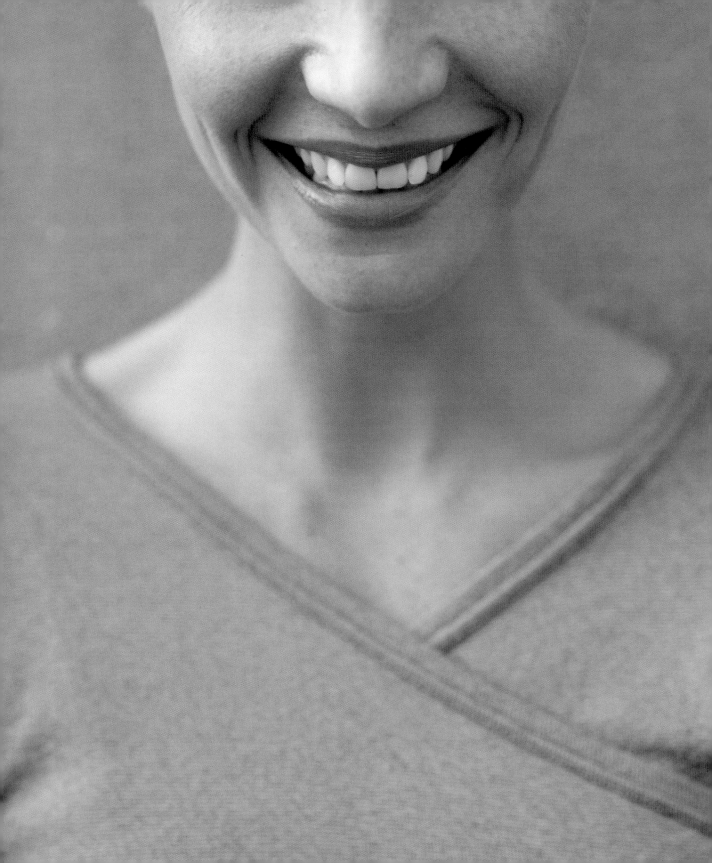

CONFIDENCE WITHOUT PLASTIC SURGERY

The men who love women love them because they are female. Take my word for it: No man worth having thinks of a woman as an object, a sculpture, a statue, or a doll. He thinks of her as a fruit: ripe, soft, natural, supple, fresh, and most important, alive.

I believe in cosmetic or corrective surgery, but I caution anyone who contemplates it impulsively. In fact, the best surgeons often advise clients to wait a few more years. Plastic surgery is great if you respect the natural proportion of your face. If not, the side effects can be devastating.

* **FOR A HAIRDRESSER**, the greatest tragedy is seeing a woman lose the natural implantation of her hair. With her new face tucked behind her ears, her hairline is off by a couple of inches. Imagine Grace Kelly's transcendent beauty if you took her hairline away.
* **I HAVE SEEN WOMEN SUBJECT THEMSELVES** to too-often-repeated peels. Their skin becomes so shiny, they look shrink-wrapped.
* **MOST PEOPLE FORGET THAT THEY CAN BE SEEN IN PROFILE.** Silicone lips may look good from the front, but can look completely artificial from the side. Beware!
* **TOO OFTEN, WHEN A LONGTIME CLIENT WALKS INTO MY SALON** after surgery, she no longer resembles the person I used to know. Her eyes are more youthful all right, but the light, the glint, the sparkle is gone. Meeting her gaze in the mirror, I suddenly become tongue-tied, unable to meet her fixed glance.

Having said that, I believe that if it is well thought out and well done, plastic surgery can help you recapture the image of who you are. But proceed with extreme caution. It's much more effective to change something small: a shot of Botox to smooth a few wrinkles rather than a chemical peel that involves more risk and recovery time.

DRY CLEAN YOUR SWEATERS AND LEAVE THEM ON HANGERS, SEALED IN THEIR PLASTIC WRAPPER, ALL SUMMER. COME OCTOBER, THEY WON'T BE WRINKLED.

22

CLEAN YOUR CLOSET BY PACKING UP THOSE VERY TRENDY PIECES OF CLOTHING YOU HARDLY WORE LAST SEASON AND GIVING THEM TO THE SALVATION ARMY OR GOODWILL.

23

REVIST THE PAINTINGS OF PAUL CÉZANNE, A NATIVE OF AIX WHO IMMORTALIZED THE COLORS OF PROVENCE IN HIS WORK. CREATE YOUR OWN BOWL-OF-FRUIT STILL-LIFE CENTERPIECE.

24

25

TAKE A LOOK AT **YOUR HAIRBRUSH.** IF THE BRISTLES ARE WORN ON THE ENDS, IT'S TIME FOR A NEW ONE. AND A NEW BRUSH FEELS GREAT ON THE SCALP.

26

IF SKI SEASON IS OVER FOR THE YEAR, PACK AWAY YOUR GEAR AND CLOTHING CAREFULLY SO IT WILL BE IN GOOD SHAPE NEXT YEAR.

27

BUY A FEW GOOD CLASSIC ITEMS FOR YOUR WARDROBE, OF THE BEST QUALITY YOU CAN AFFORD. STERLING FAVORITES: STRAIGHT BLACK PANTS, A CARDIGAN, DRIVING MOCCASINS. WEAR THEM WITH A PONYTAIL.

Kiss and tell: Let me be the champion of the natural woman.

One exception to these cautionary tales is cosmetic dentistry. I've seen smiles and faces transformed through corrective or whitening procedures, and they can actually help preserve the shape of your face. They can also take off years—if only because you'll want to flash that smile more often!

HOW TO SHINE LIKE A STAR

If you're someone who's not especially comfortable with a lot of ornamentation or elaborate preparations before a night in the spotlight, the California take on glamour may be just right for you. Here's simplicity in its purest and prettiest form. For anything less than a gala nighttime event (see page 231 for more on that), less truly is more. Maybe a silk slipdress and a bit of lipgloss. Or a simple sleeveless sheath with your long straight hair held in place by a pretty ornament. Wear fabulous sandals or dainty mules. And never forget an elegant little evening bag.

Going all out in Hollywood requires you to be prepared.

* **START BY PUTTING ON THE GLITZ** inside before you put it outside: In other words, get a massage, a sea-salt scrub (for that baby skin to go with the bare look), a manicure, and a pedicure. Feeling relaxed and confident is about the most efficient thing you can do to look like a million dollars, and in Los Angeles bare skin is the most essential accessory there is for a nighttime look.

* **THE STYLE OF YOUR HAIR** is at least as critical as the style of your dress, but beware of complicated dos. In fact, the more glamorous the event you attend, the simpler your coiffure should be. Stars have learned that with lights, cameras, microphones, limos, red carpets, designer gowns, jewels, and other celebrities everywhere, simple really stands out.

* **HAIR ORNAMENTS ARE JEWELRY.** Think twice before mixing them with other pieces.
* **DON'T WEAR BLACK!** Unless your gown has an amazing shape or silhouette, no one will notice you. Flaunt it with an eye-catching dress, but don't skimp on the quality. There is nothing worse than a stunning outfit with cheap-looking craftsmanship, particularly seams that pucker.
* **APPLY JUST ENOUGH MAKEUP** to focus the attention on your face and your natural beauty; let it quietly speak for itself.
* **FOR DAYTIME GLAMOUR,** wear only jewelry with a meaning: an heirloom cross; the beautiful ring that was a gift from your sweetheart's grandmother; or, dangling on a chain, a crystal or some precious stone that has spiritual or emotional meaning. Save the chunky stuff for nocturnal revelry.
* **BY ALL MEANS, WEAR FABULOUS SUNGLASSES,** but if you do, be ready to eliminate other accessories. Get rid of your silk scarf (too cliché). Take off your gold jewelry (too obvious). Don't even consider wearing your red gloves (please!).
* **NIGHT OR DAY,** there is one rule for pantyhose and stockings: If you notice them, it's ugly. Your hosiery should be barely visible, just a haze over your leg.

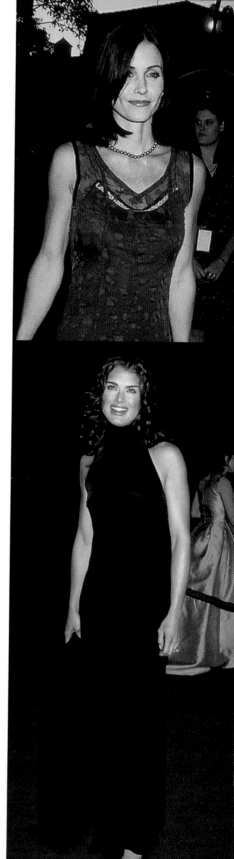

TOP: I LOVE COURTENEY COX ARQUETTE'S DARK HAIR, FAIR SKIN AND BLUE EYES. IT'S AN UNCOMMON COMBINATION. SHE LOOKS GREAT WITH A STRAIGHT BOB OR LONGER HAIR WITH BANGS. **BOTTOM:** BROOKE SHIELDS IS A GORGEOUS WOMAN AND A PERFECT EXAMPLE OF SOMEONE WHO KNOWS THAT SIMPLICITY IS KEY TO GREAT STYLE.

28 EVEN ON CASUAL DAYS, **IRON YOUR KHAKIS AND T-SHIRTS,** FOR QUIET ELEGANCE.

29 **THROW OUT THOSE WEIRD CREAMS** THAT OVER-PROMISED AND NEVER PERFORMED. GET BACK TO BASICS

30 TAKE A MENTAL VACATION: DON'T SPEAK FOR AT LEAST TWO HOURS.

31 **DON'T JUDGE PEOPLE BY THEIR RELATIVES.**

SUNGLASSES

Sunglasses are instant chic. They convey attitude and confidence, sophistication and style. They should never look weak, timid, or ordinary.

* TAKE THE TIME TO PICK OUT the right pair of sunglasses. If you love them, you'll wear them more than any other accessory.

* GREAT SUNGLASSES are almost like a great haircut—they're always part of your look.

* SUNGLASSES WITH TOO MUCH GOLD ornamentation on them—no matter what the logo is—look cheap.

* BLACK FRAMES work on almost every skin tone.

* SPEND AS MUCH AS YOU CAN afford on the quality of the lens. Cheap sunglasses will make you squint and increase your chance of getting wrinkles.

* WRAP-AROUND SUNGLASSES give you a sense of security. But beware: Though you may enjoy feeling like a movie star traveling incognito, you will look terribly aloof.

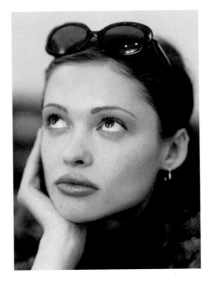

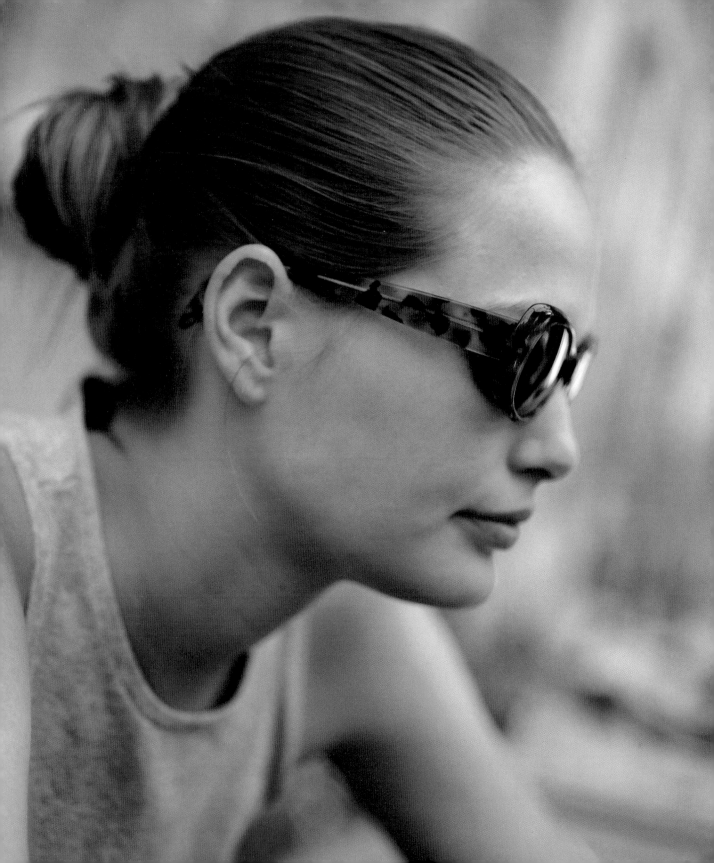

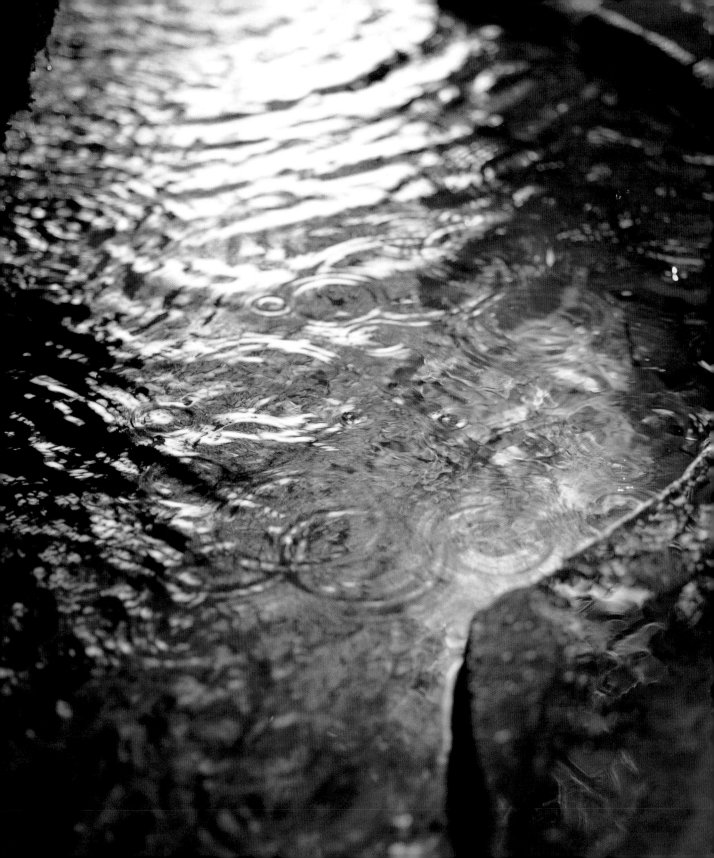

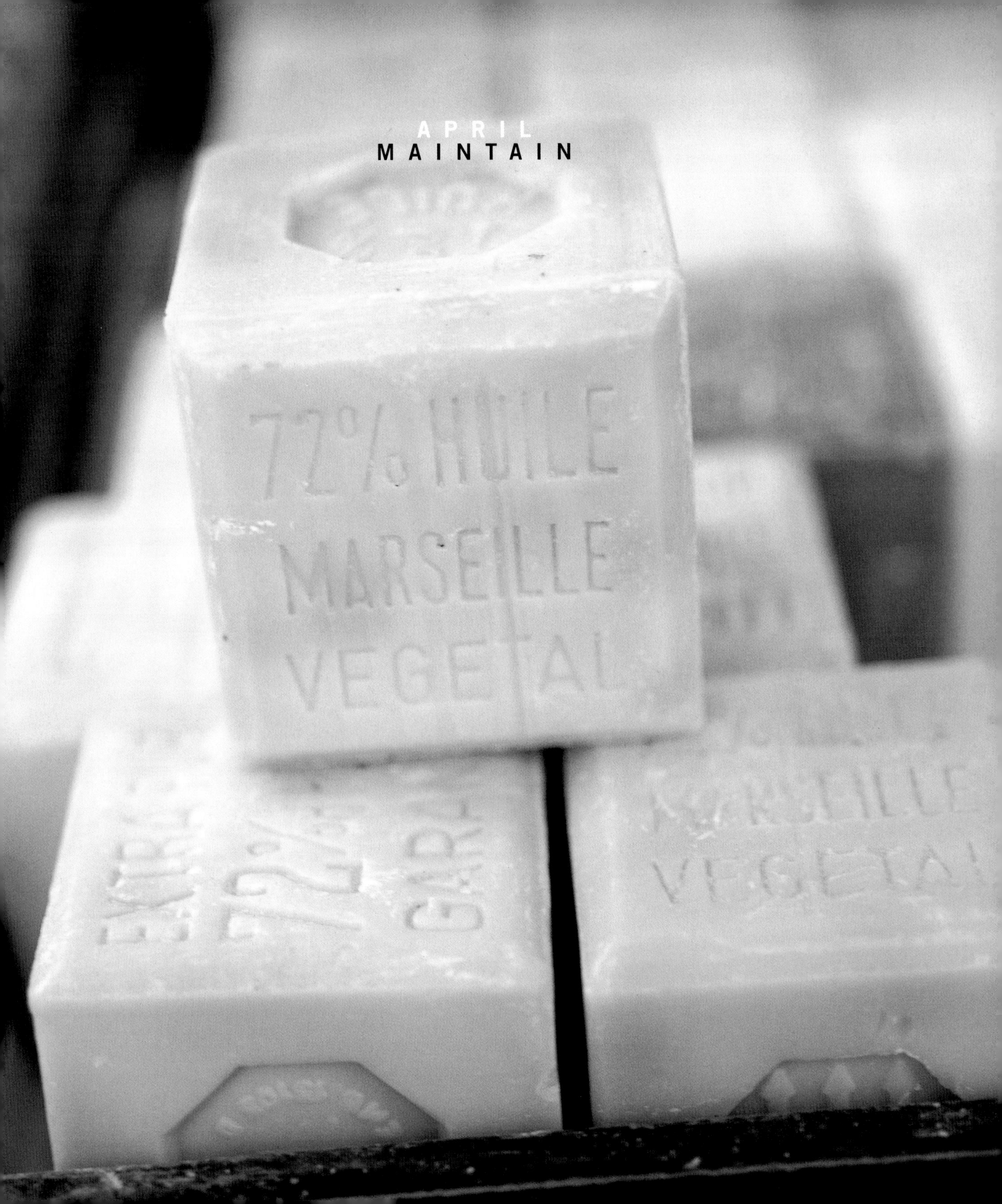

1 AS A QUICK MEDITATION EXERCISE, INHALE DEEPLY, SMILE, AND CLOSE YOUR EYES AT THE SAME TIME. SLOWLY EXHALE.

2 STEAM SOME PENCIL-THIN ASPARAGUS SPEARS AND COVER THEM WITH LEMON, FRESH-GRATED PARMESAN CHEESE, BLACK PEPPER, AND NOTHING ELSE.

3 A BARE TOP IN A WARM, DEEP TONE IS GLAMOROUS FOR EARLY SPRING EVENINGS. BRING A SHAWL.

I admire the way women in Aix dress on rainy days. Instead of letting the gray sky affect their mood, they react by wearing more sophisticated clothes. If the temperature is mild, they go singing in the rain under a big umbrella in bright light outfits that flutter in the wind. If it's cold, they put on stretch pants, a cashmere turtleneck, tall black boots, and throw an oiled Barbour on top of it all.

In April, you never know whether it's going to be warm or cold outside. Spring is always fashionably late, to give you time to get ready for what is probably the biggest seasonal change of the year—the re-awakening of nature. Buds take their time pampering themselves before blooming, and so should you. Use the month of April to revive your senses and reactivate your body. Find a new fragrance. Sign up for massage therapy. Buy daffodils and ranunculus by the bucket. Splurge on a new handbag. Get a facial. Flush away mental toxins.

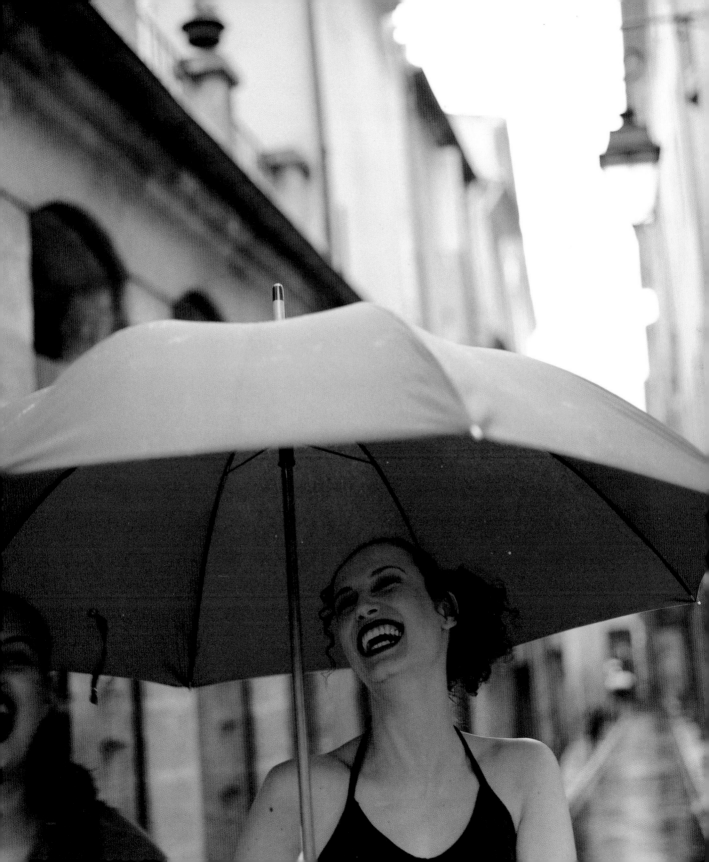

LEAVE THE HOUSE DRESSED AS IF TODAY WERE A SPECIAL DAY. YOU NEVER KNOW. SPRING IS IN THE AIR!

4

HAVE A SEA-SALT BODY SCRUB OR A SEAWEED WRAP TO ELIMINATE TOXINS.

5

DON'T BE FOOLED BY COOL TEMPERATURES. THE SUN IS ALREADY STRONGER AND A HAT OR A GOOD SUNSCREEN IS A MUST.

6

You owe it to yourself to book a couple of day spa sessions. Choose a spa first and foremost for its relaxing atmosphere. Music, running water, pastel colors, diffused light, fluffy towels, fruits, scents . . . these elements are as much a part of the holistic process as the massages, the body scrubs, and the herbal tea wraps. Take my word for it: The beauty of the decor can lower your blood pressure and calm your nerves faster than an exotic Shirodhara treatment or a lengthy Pancha Karma therapy session.

If you don't have time to go to a spa, take a few minutes every day after your regular shower or bath to massage your extremities, your fingers, your toes, your ears, your scalp. Use a wet washcloth, a loofah glove, or some gentle exfoliating cream to polish your skin and drive the tensions out of your body.

SALON TREATMENTS

There are dozens of spa treatments available today, ranging from the exotic to the traditional. Entire spas are devoted to Ayurvedic practice, aromatherapy, Eastern European methods, and more. If I was to recommend just one treatment to sluff off the old, prepare for the new, it would be a massage or a facial. In Europe no woman goes longer than a month without receiving one or both of these refining treatments and it's a practice American women should adopt.

RIGHT: GOING TO A SPA SHOULD ALWAYS BE A LUXURIOUS EXPERIENCE, WITH A TOUCH OF LAST YEAR IN MARIENBAD.

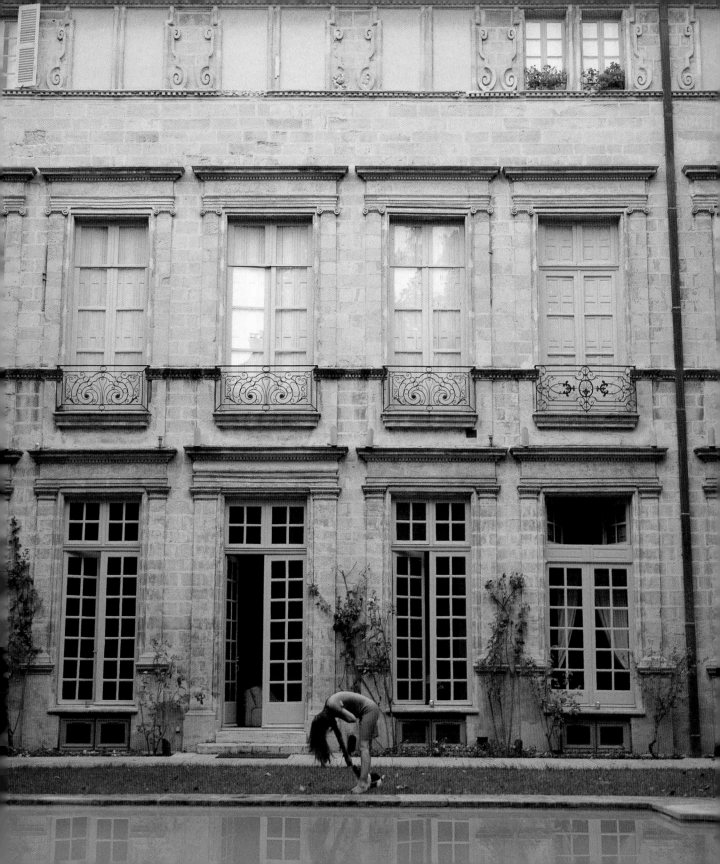

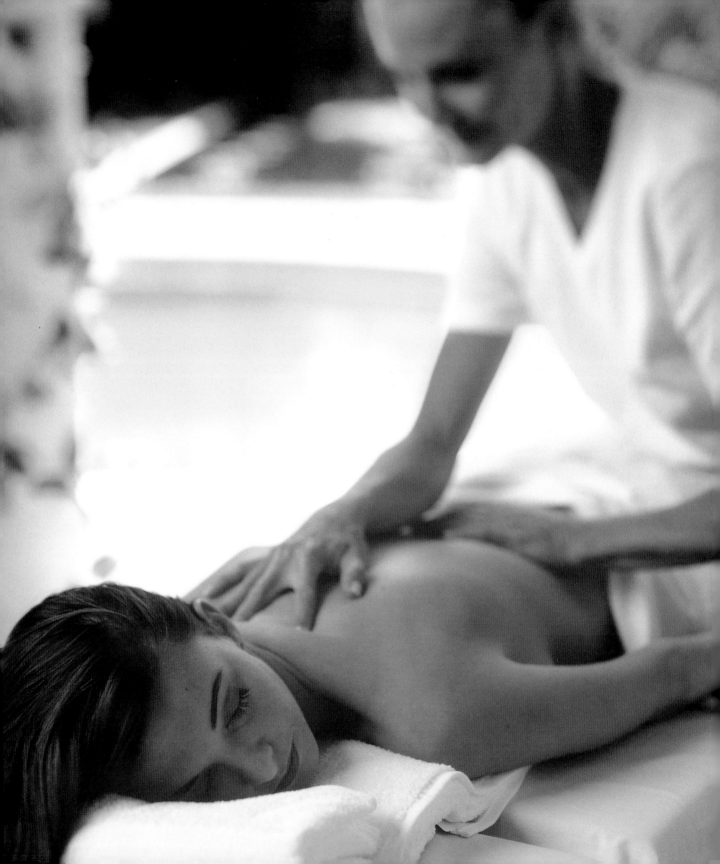

MASSAGE

Massage is relaxing, but it's also energizing, particularly if you combine different techniques: Swedish massage, which kneads the muscles in the classic, rubdown style; Shiatsu, which focuses on Eastern acupressure points; and lately, Thai massage, which involves more actual stretching and moving of your muscles. To get the most of a massage, any massage, you can't be anxious beforehand. You have to know what to expect.

* **WHAT KIND OF MASSAGE IS IT?** For a Shiatsu massage, for instance, you'd want to wear loose clothing; for a Swedish massage, you will be expected to take all your clothes off.
* **GO TO A REPUTABLE SALON:** Follow a friend's or a magazine's recommendation, or go to a day spa in a hotel you love. Once you're there, everything—slippers, sheets, bathrobes, showers—should be clean and fresh.
* **DECIDE IN ADVANCE** whether you want a man or a woman to do the massage, and let the receptionist know when you book the appointment.
* **TALK WITH THE MASSAGE THERAPIST** to determine what kind of pressure you like best, or perhaps what type of music is more relaxing to you. But beyond that, no small talk. You need to be able to zone out.
* **DON'T GET A MASSAGE IF** you're planning to go out later, or do anything requiring all your pep and enthusiasm. Though you feel great, you don't want to squander your energy on extroverted pursuits.

FACIALS

A facial should be an effective yet pleasurable experience. Don't trust just anyone with your face. Try to find an aesthetician who believes in the scientific approach—someone who was trained in the tradition of European spas, not a beautician. Skin is a vital organ and should be treated as care.

Before a facial, you want to talk with the aesthetician in the same way you discuss your health with a doctor. She should ask about your skin type,

Mirrors should reflect a little before throwing back images.
—JEAN COCTEAU

7

REPLACE YOUR FOLDING UMBRELLA WITH A STURDY FULL-SIZED ONE WITH AN INTERESTING HANDLE.

8

SEE A DERMATOLOGIST TO MAKE SURE YOUR SKIN CAN BE SAFELY EXPOSED TO THE SUN.

9

10 HAVE YOU MADE AN APPOINTMENT FOR A **DENTAL CLEANING** RECENTLY?

11 SIGN UP FOR A SESSION **WITH A PERSONAL TRAINER** TO MAKE SURE THAT YOUR FITNESS ROUTINE IS ON TARGET.

12 ROLL UP SPARE CHANGE AND **DONATE THE PROCEEDS TO A CHARITY**.

whether you sleep enough, and whether you're allergic or sensitive to any foods. Discuss the effect stress has on your skin. This first interview will ensure that your facial is customized, and that the treatment will target your particular needs. Be sure your facial involves these components:

* **BEFORE CLEANSING YOUR SKIN,** a good aesthetician should give you a soothing upper-body massage to relax you, erase the tensions from your face, and stimulate your skin.
* **SHE SHOULD EXPLAIN TO YOU** what products she intends to use—and why. For example, orange extract is good for closing pores, yet too much of it can cause skin flare-ups.
* **SHE SHOULD USE ONLY COTTON,** sponges, and soft brushes to remove impurities—no scary-looking tools.
* **SHE SHOULD STAY AWAY FROM FRAGRANCED PRODUCTS** and coarse exfoliators that could induce allergic reactions.
* **FINALLY, AS A TREAT,** she should give you a scalp and hand massage.

Your face may be a bit red when you leave the salon. Don't be alarmed; ice applications can reduce the redness and slight swelling if need be, but within a couple of hours your skin will be soft and radiant.

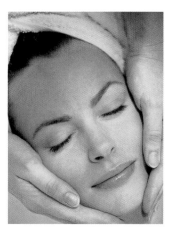

AT HOME MAINTENANCE

Hair, like skin, needs to be pampered in order to stay in shape. Too often, unfortunately, the nurturing products designed to go on your hair end up on your scalp, where they stick like glue, or even worse, down the drain, where the nutrients are washed away. This is true of shampoos, conditioners, rinses, creams, masks, sprays, or gels. To avoid wasting hair products, never apply them directly on your head: Pour into your hands first, and only then apply to your hair. It's one more step—I know, you are in a rush—but it allows you to control how much product is applied and, most important, where it goes, whether on the tips or the roots of your hair.

It's surprising how difficult it is to understand—and memorize—the claims and the directions on the bottles. Should you use gel for short hair or long hair? At the roots or on the ends? What about mousse? What's the difference? In the salon, we're careful to explain exactly what different products are supposed to do, and how they might work with different hairstyles and types. The secret of good maintenance is to use the right products correctly. Once you understand how different products should work, it becomes so much easier to nurture and style your hair.

GETTING THE MOST FROM YOUR SHAMPOO

I do think most people look best if they wash their hair every day. The exception would be people with extremely thick or frizzy hair, which can, in some cases, be washed and blown out every five days and not touched in between. A great shampoo will accommodate daily washing, and it should leave your hair shiny, bouncy, and healthy-looking.

✳ **SHAMPOO DOESN'T DRY OUT YOUR HAIR;** heat from blow-dryers, hot rollers, curling irons, and straightening irons does. If your hair is getting dry and fragile, don't stop washing it, just ease up on the heat appliances.

TIME TO CHANGE YOUR BEDSPREAD FROM QUILTED FLANNEL OR DOWN TO COTTON PIQUÉ.

13

REMEMBER TO **DRINK TONS OF WATER,** WHETHER OR NOT YOU ARE THIRSTY.

14

ALWAYS APPLY STYLING PRODUCTS TO **TOWEL-DRIED HAIR**; IF THE HAIR IS TOO WET, THE PRODUCTS WILL BE DILUTED AND LESS EFFECTIVE.

15

16

ALWAYS KEEP A FULL-SIZE UMBRELLA IN THE TRUNK OF YOUR CAR SO YOU CAN ARRIVE AT DESTINATIONS SPOTLESS AND DRY.

16

DEVISE A FILING SYSTEM TO ORGANIZE ARTICLES AND PHOTOS YOU'VE BEEN SAVING.

17

DON'T SKIMP ON HOSIERY AND STOCKINGS. CHEAP ONES CAN REALLY DETRACT FROM YOUR OVERALL LOOK.

18

* **SHAMPOO SHOULD FEEL GREAT** and smell wonderful in the shower, but it shouldn't leave a heavy scent on your hair once it's rinsed out.
* **MAKE SURE YOUR HAIR IS REALLY WET** before you put in any shampoo. If it isn't completely and absolutely wet to the roots, the shampoo won't flow through the hair. When you try to rinse it out, some of it will stick to hair that wasn't wet to begin with. The result is a mane that's dull or even flaky due to shampoo residues.
* **WHEN YOU APPLY THE SHAMPOO**, don't just put it all on the top of your head. Apply a little bit at the forehead, crown, temples, and the nape of the neck. Then use a comb to distribute the shampoo through the hair.
* **WHEN YOU RINSE YOUR HAIR** (of shampoo but also of conditioner), first use warm water, then switch to the coldest water you can bear. Warm water opens the hair shaft, and cold water closes it. The result is much shinier hair. True, few of us relish a cold shower first thing in the morning (or any time) but tell yourself that the colder the water, the shinier your hair. You will see a difference.

CONDITIONERS AND RINSES

Most hair needs conditioning as regularly as it needs washing. Even very oily hair can be dry and brittle at the ends, and conditioners can restore its flexibility and prevent breakage. They also help hair stand up to the assaults of brushes, heat appliances, and environmental factors like sun, pollution, and cold. The right conditioning product feels right, smells great, and leaves your hair feeling and looking better than it did before.

Use either a rinse or conditioner, but never the two together. Although both products act as detanglers and improve the shine of your hair they counter each other's action. Rinses strip your hair of all impurities while conditioners coat it with nutrients. Rinses are best for oily hair, but not appropriate for colored hair. They can make the color fade faster. Conditioners, in contrast, add weight, body, and moisture to dry hair.

So use a conditioner, keeping these tips in mind:

* **NEVER APPLY THE PRODUCT TO YOUR SCALP,** unless you have a dry scalp. Keep it out of the roots; it weighs hair down.
* **COMB YOUR HAIR WITH A WIDE-TOOTH COMB,** then rinse with cold water as you continue to comb. Besides closing the hair shaft, the cold water also stimulates circulation in the scalp, giving the hair even more shine.

CONDITIONING MASKS

Once a month, or even once a week if your hair is very dry or damaged, treat your hair to some really intensive conditioning. I remember women along the Riviera slicking their hair back with coconut oil before they went out onto the beach for the day. The principle is a very good one: Heat helps the oil absorb into the hair shaft, so it can really saturate the hair.

Oil, of course, is a little messy for most people. A hair mask, which will generally incorporate nutrients and other conditioners that will benefit your hair, is a good alternative.

You don't have to wash your hair first, but do apply masks (or shea butter) to wet hair. Coat your hair with the mask and let it remain for at least 20 minutes, or for the whole day if you want. Comb back into a ponytail, and leave your hair uncovered, or wear a scarf if you prefer. The longer you leave the mask, the shinier, healthier, and bouncier your hair will be. Afterward, wash your hair, but don't apply a rinse or conditioner.

LEAVE-IN CONDITIONERS

An entirely different class of conditioning product, these are formulated to be applied to wet or dry hair in place of regular conditioner but not rinsed out. Consider one of these products if:

*YOUR HAIR IS VERY DRY and needs an added bit of moisture even after using a regular conditioner.

*KNOTS AND TANGLES are a problem for your hair (especially if it's long).

*LEAVE-IN CONDITIONING SPRITZES are also a godsend for children's fine hair.

19 **FIND A COLORFUL RAINCOAT** TO MAKE APRIL SHOWERS FUN.

20 **CHANGE YOUR LIGHTBULBS** FROM FROSTED TO CLEAR TO MAKE YOUR HOME MORE SPARKLING.

21 **WRITE A REAL LETTER TO A FRIEND** YOU HAVEN'T HAD TIME TO CALL IN MONTHS.

SHEA BUTTER

For centuries, shea butter has been prized for its nourishing effects on skin and hair, and it's been a fixture in French pharmacies for as long as I can remember. It smells like a tropical vacation, and it's just an incredible moisturizer, one of those examples of an ancient remedy that far surpasses anything scientists have devised. It's great to mix with gel, because it softens up the gel's texture in your hair, but you still get a bit of hold. I mix it into practically everything: my body scrub, hair masks, and more. Look for it in lip balm, soap, body lotion. Use it full strength as a hair mask. You'll love the results.

THE NATURAL GOLDEN TAN

Many women are afraid to try self-tanners—they think they streak, they won't look natural, they are bad for your skin. Not so: Self-tanners today, for the most part, are enriched with vitamins and nutrients. And they give the appearance of an even, realistic tan if applied correctly. Take the time to do it right, and I know you'll be thrilled with the results. Or ask at your salon; many offer self-tanning treatments.

* **BEFORE YOU BUY A SELF-TANNER**, unscrew the cap and take a sniff to make sure you like the fragrance.
* **EXFOLIATE IN THE SHOWER**, using a lightweight body scrub that gently polishes rough, dry skin and prepares it for an application of self-bronzer. But be sure to use a product with moisturizing benefits, one specifically formulated to leave you feeling soft, silky, and glowing.
* **TOWEL OFF THOROUGHLY.**
* **APPLY THE SELF-TANNER**, lots of it. The single most important way to make a self-tan look good is to use enough of it, so make sure you really get full coverage. Using more self-tanner won't make the tan any darker, it will simply blend better. Blend it as thoroughly as you can.
* **DON'T TAN IN PLACES** that the sun would never normally reach, the lighter underside of your arm, for instance.

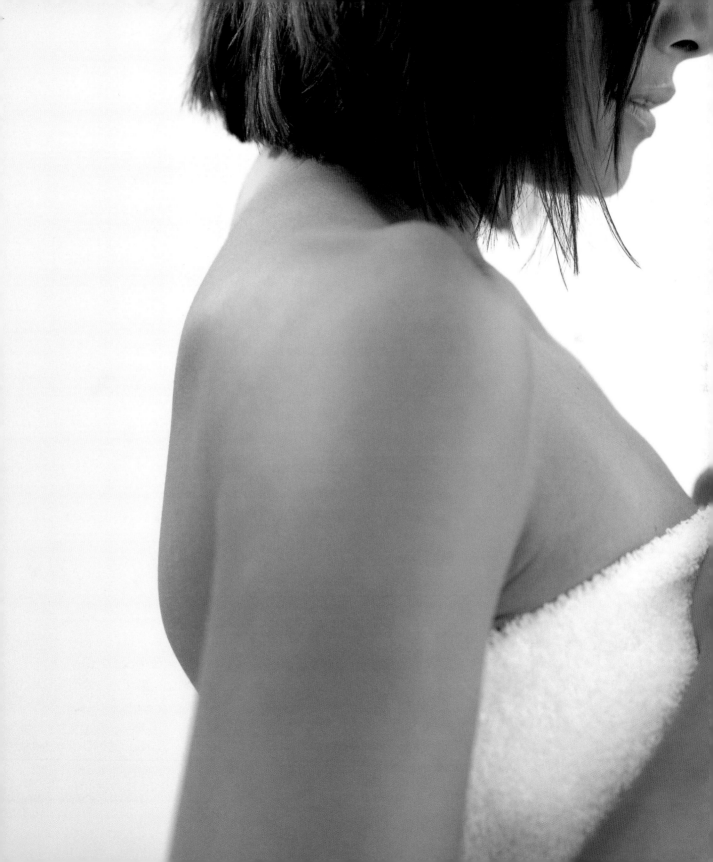

22

Everyday I simplify something, because everyday I learn something.

—COCO CHANEL

23

ASK FRIENDS WHO GO TO FRANCE TO BRING YOU BACK SAVON DE MARSEILLES SOAP. MADE WITH OLIVE OIL, IT HAS MOISTURING *AND* ASTRINGENT PROPERTIES THAT WORK WONDERS AGAINST BLEMISHES.

24

TRY A MUD BATH TO REPLENISH THE MOISTURE OF YOUR SKIN.

* **SELF-TANNERS WORK JUST AS WELL ON THE FACE AND NECK** as the rest of the body, though you'll want to blend carefully at the hairline, and avoid getting self-tanner on the brows.
* **ONCE YOU'VE REALLY WORKED IT IN**, wash your hands—you don't want to leave it on your palms.
* **ROUGH SKIN**, like your elbows, anklebones, or the tips of your toes, will absorb more self-tanner than the rest of your body, so smooth a wet washcloth or tissue over rough areas immediately after you've finished blending, to wipe off the self-tanner in those spots.
* **PUT A DOT OF SELF-TANNER** on the back of one hand; rub it against the back of your other hand. Your hands will be tan; your palms will not.
* **IF YOU DON'T HAVE THE TIME** or inclination to wait for the tanner to dry, slip on something dark and washable.

Self-tanners work to stain the outer layers of your skin, producing a golden tone. You get the same effect as if you were lying in the sun for an afternoon, without being bombarded by harmful ultraviolet rays.

If you tan easily, chances are your self-tanner will create a deep, luxurious tan. If you stay relatively pale during the summer months, you will get just a hint of bronze. So don't worry: one application of self-tanning lotion will not change the nature of your skin—you won't wake up looking like some exotic clone of your original self.

Dark tans are no longer required to be considered chic or elegant. The goal of self-tanning is to make you look healthy, not colorful. Coco Chanel first championed the light tawny glow in the twenties, and today a discreet tan still conveys a sense of relaxation, of being well-rested and at ease. Clients in my Los Angeles salon have perfected the art of looking ever-so-slightly tanned, the result of year-round outdoor living. They maintain a radiant complexion with weekly applications of self-tanner. As a result, they need less makeup and look naturally pretty.

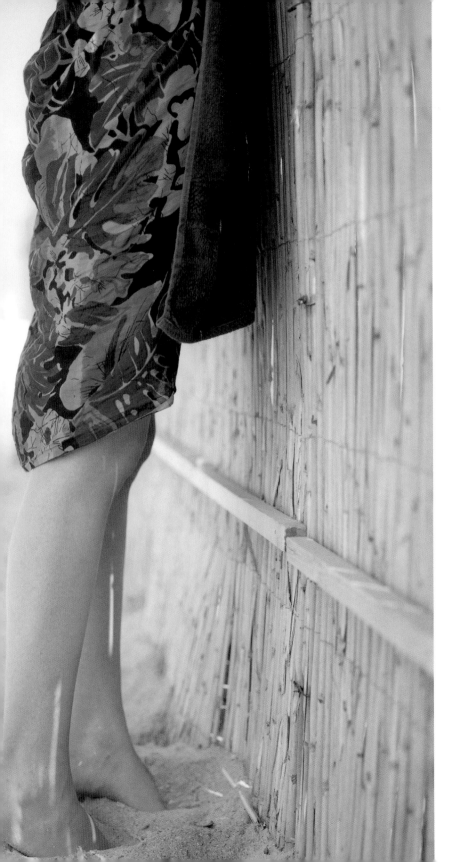

HOW TO WRAP A PAREO

Originally from the South Pacific, pareos became fashionable in chic French resort towns in the 1930s. The look was adopted by women eager to emulate the pencil-thin wrapped outfits of Mademoiselle Chanel.

Pareo fabric is light yet opaque. It dries quickly and doesn't wrinkle easily. The patterns are often bold batik motifs in tangerine, mandarin, mint, cerulean blue, turquoise.

* WRAP THE PAREO around you so the top hits you at the waist.

* HOLD THE TOP of each end out in front, at waist level.

* START TO TWIST the two ends, and keep twisting until you can't twist anymore.

* TUCK THE ENDS IN and under around your waist.

* WEAR WITH A STRAPLESS tube top or with a simple little T-shirt in a solid color.

* FLAT SANDALS, black ballerina shoes, or cotton espadrilles (or bare feet) complete the look. Never wear a pareo with high heels!

25 NOW IS THE TIME TO **SWITCH TO A LIGHTER SPRING FRAGRANCE.**

26 IF YOU CAN'T GET AWAY, PUT ON CARIBBEAN MUSIC, MIX UP A MAI TAI, SIT BY A SUNNY WINDOW, AND DREAM.

27 **SPLURGE ON A NEW PAIR OF SHOES**—AND A NEW BELT WHILE YOU'RE AT IT.

THE ULTIMATE SPA TREATMENT: GET TROPICAL!

By the time April comes, I'm so tired of cold weather that I nearly always sneak off for a tropical vacation. It's the perfect time to go: The winter crowds are gone, the weather's ideal, and I'm in the mood! I love the fact that in just four hours I can go from the dead of winter to a tropical resort without time change or jet lag.

Choose a resort, or better yet an island, with a small town nearby. I am partial to St. Barthélemy for its French culture, its little cafés, its sailboats, its blue sky, and its easy pace. Wherever you go, make sure you can start your day with mangoes, café au lait, and croissants, then move quickly to the beach. Your daytime wardrobe should consist of nothing more than a pareo and a T-shirt over your bathing suit, with a hat and a big straw bag in which you tuck away your daily essentials: a pair of sunglasses, hair conditioning spray with built-in sun protection (especially important if you color your hair), a wide-tooth comb, a large barrette or elastic headband to pull your hair back, sunscreen, a bottle of water, towels, and a great book. This tropical look has tried-and-true allure and attitude.

If you are not the sort to while away hours at the beach, pick a tropical resort with great shopping. All you want is a couple of small exclusive boutiques, with one-of-a-kind offerings. In St. Barth, my favorite spot is a shop called La Marine that sells striped T-shirts and French espadrilles. After shopping, I stop for a pastis or a *citron pressé*. If it's Thursday, I have dinner at L'Escale, where fresh mussels are on the menu. Otherwise, there's the fabulous Maya, another French eatery with a most romantic view.

RIGHT: LOTS OF WATER ON WINTER-DRY SKIN CAN DEHYDRATE YOU. BE SURE TO USE PLENTY OF MOISTURIZER AND, OF COURSE, SUNSCREEN.

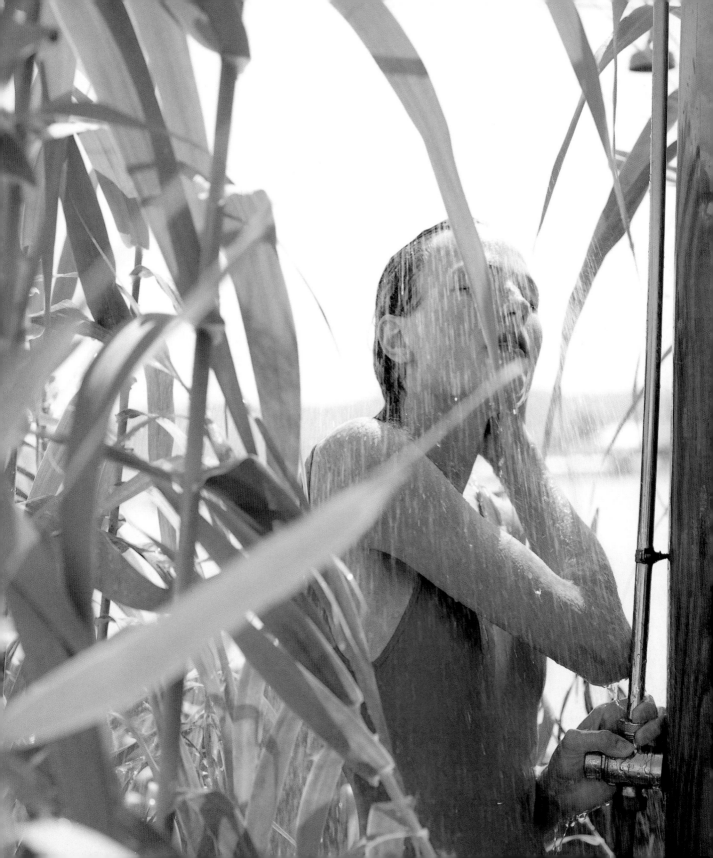

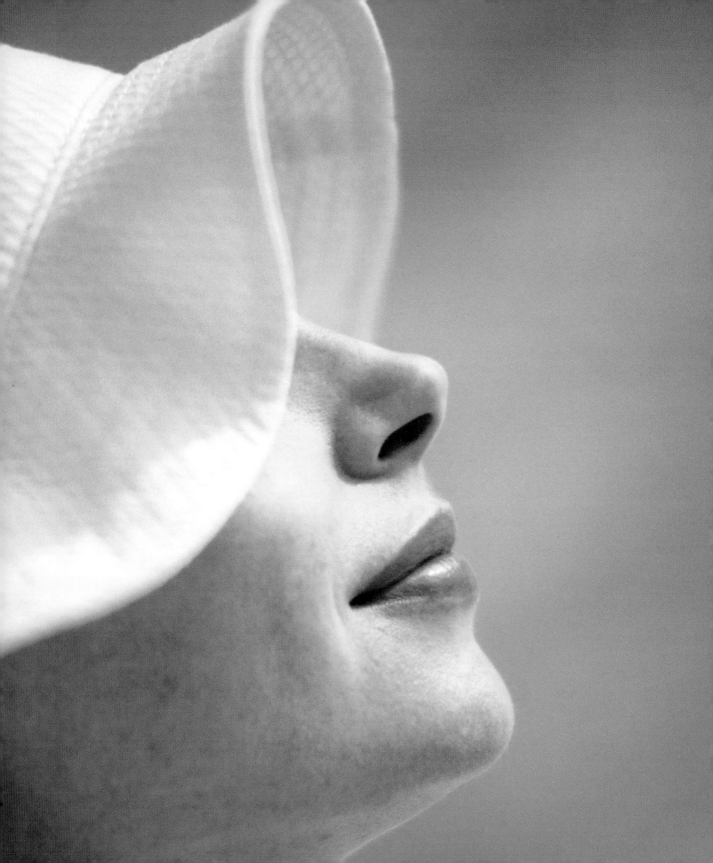

HATS

One of the delights of going to a tropical resort is rediscovering the pleasure of wearing a hat. Although hats no longer play a major role in fashion, they can be ultra chic, especially for sun protection. Next time you are on vacation, practice looking at the world from beneath the brim of a straw Panama. You'll have a more relaxed, more open perspective on all you survey.

Here are a few rules for carrying off a hat in style, whether you are in the tropics or back home.

* GO WITH LIGHT, and go with soft. You don't want anything heavy on your head. Fabrics like cotton, linen, or microfiber are perfect. So is straw.

* TO AVOID HAT HAIR, wear a hat that lets air through, and take it off every few hours. Brush your hair back before you put the hat on, and when you take it off, flip your head upside down and brush downward a few times.

* HATS WITH A BILL, like baseball caps, are fabulous for the beach, not to mention driving in an open convertible, playing tennis, hiking, or boating.

* HATS AND SUNGLASSES are perfect together. The combination is very Hollywood.

* WEARING YOUR HAT slightly askew gives you a jaunty look.

* WHEN WEARING A BERET, pull a few strands of hair in front of your face for a softer style.

* FOR MEN, wearing a hat at all times is rude. A hat is like a coat: Take it off when you go inside.

HUG LOVED ONES EVERYDAY. **28**

PEONIES ARE MY FAVORITE FLOWER, AND THEY SHOW UP AT FLORISTS TOWARD THE END OF APRIL. MASS THEM IN VASES ALL OVER YOUR HOUSE. **29**

RELAX AT THE END OF THE DAY WITH WARM COMPRESSES ON YOUR NECK AND SHOULDERS. **30**

WHAT TO AVOID

Pregnant women are famous for wanting to eat ice cream with pickles at three in the morning. I will always envy them this privilege. On the other hand, some impulses should be curbed:

* The urge to cut your hair very, very short. Now is not the time for a radical change; you'll probably regret it. Save the style transformations for later. A refreshing trim, a sleek ponytail, or wearing your hair up in a chignon are better solutions for now.

* The wish to lie down and eat bonbons all day long. Sorry. Forget it. Don't stop exercising. Speak to your doctor about how to tailor your routine as your pregnancy progresses, but keep up your good habits.

* No matter how many kinks you feel at the end of the day, now is not the time to soak in a hot tub, take a steam bath, get into a sauna, or have an herbal wrap. Heat treatments are not recommended during pregnancy.

BEAUTY MAINTENANCE
FOR PREGNANT WOMEN

We can all learn about real beauty from watching pregnant women. Probably because the prospect of a birth is such a happy event, mothers-to-be are more radiant, more peaceful, more confident than other women.

In Europe, most women wear body-skimming clothes to show off their new shape when they're expecting. In America, I find most pregnant women try to hide their midriff. Get rid of your loose tunics and empire-waisted dresses. Instead, wear body-contouring clothes in dark colors that enhance your shape. It's very chic to be pregnant and flaunt it by wearing outfits that are just as stylish as your regular wardrobe.

Too many women spend their pregnancy worrying about their weight. Why not forget about it for nine months? This is the one time in your life when extra pounds look good on you. And think of all the great trade-offs: your newly glowing skin, your luxuriously thick hair, and your right to take as many catnaps on the sofa as you want without feeling guilty.

However, the glow of pregnancy won't replace routine maintenance to keep your skin fresh, your hair swinging. Keep your regular schedule of beauty treatments or add some new ones. There was a big hair color scare several years ago (a study seemed to show that hair color might affect a growing fetus), which was later disproved. Nonetheless, many of my clients play it safe and ease up on their color. One good solution is to get highlights that don't actually come in contact with the scalp.

* A great haircut will make you feel trim.
* A facial will completely refresh you.
* A scrub with fresh ginger can help ease nausea.
* A light massage will relax you.
* A pedicure with reflexology will soothe you from head to toe.

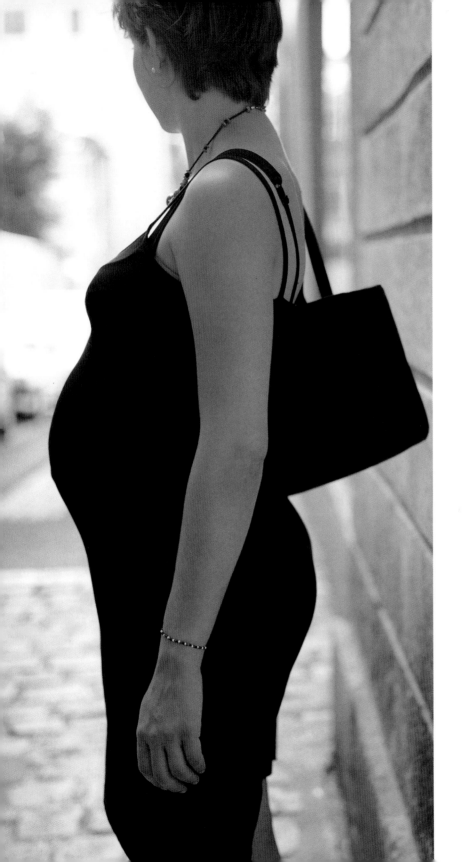

PREGNANCY AND HAIR LOSS

Many of my clients have problems with hair loss right after giving birth. This can be alarming, but fortunately, it's temporary. Just hang in there. Get regular cuts, and experiment with texturizing balms to play up shine as much as possible. If you get those little "bangs" around your forehead—they're caused by new hair growth—use a gel or cream to push them back, or cut real bangs to mask them. With frequent trims, they will eventually catch up with the rest of your hair.

Once you've had the baby, remember to stick to some of your old de-stressing routines: Take a little time out for yourself to feel beautiful. It is so important—for you, for your marriage, for your baby.

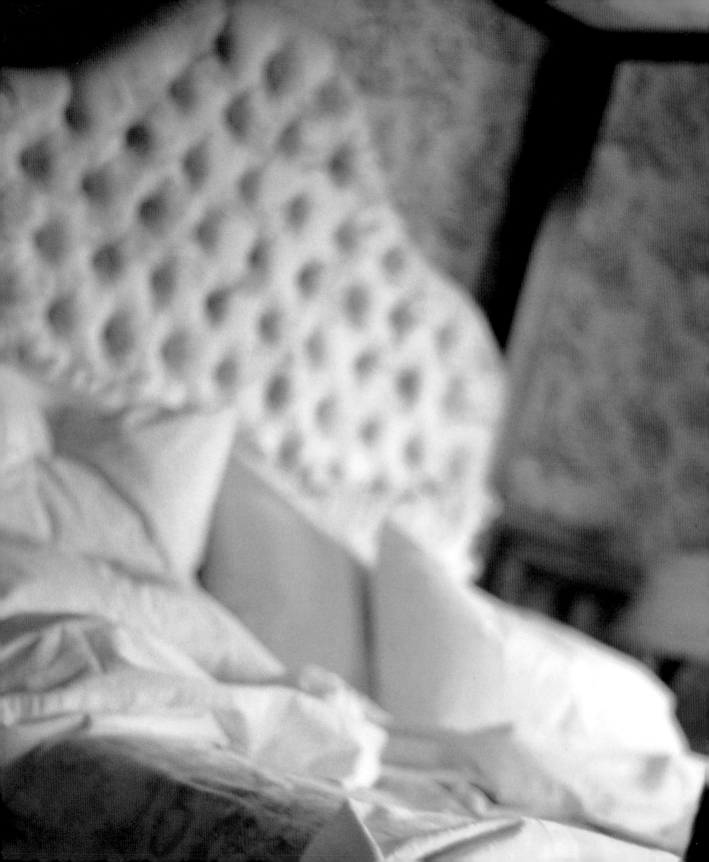

MAY
SENSUALITY

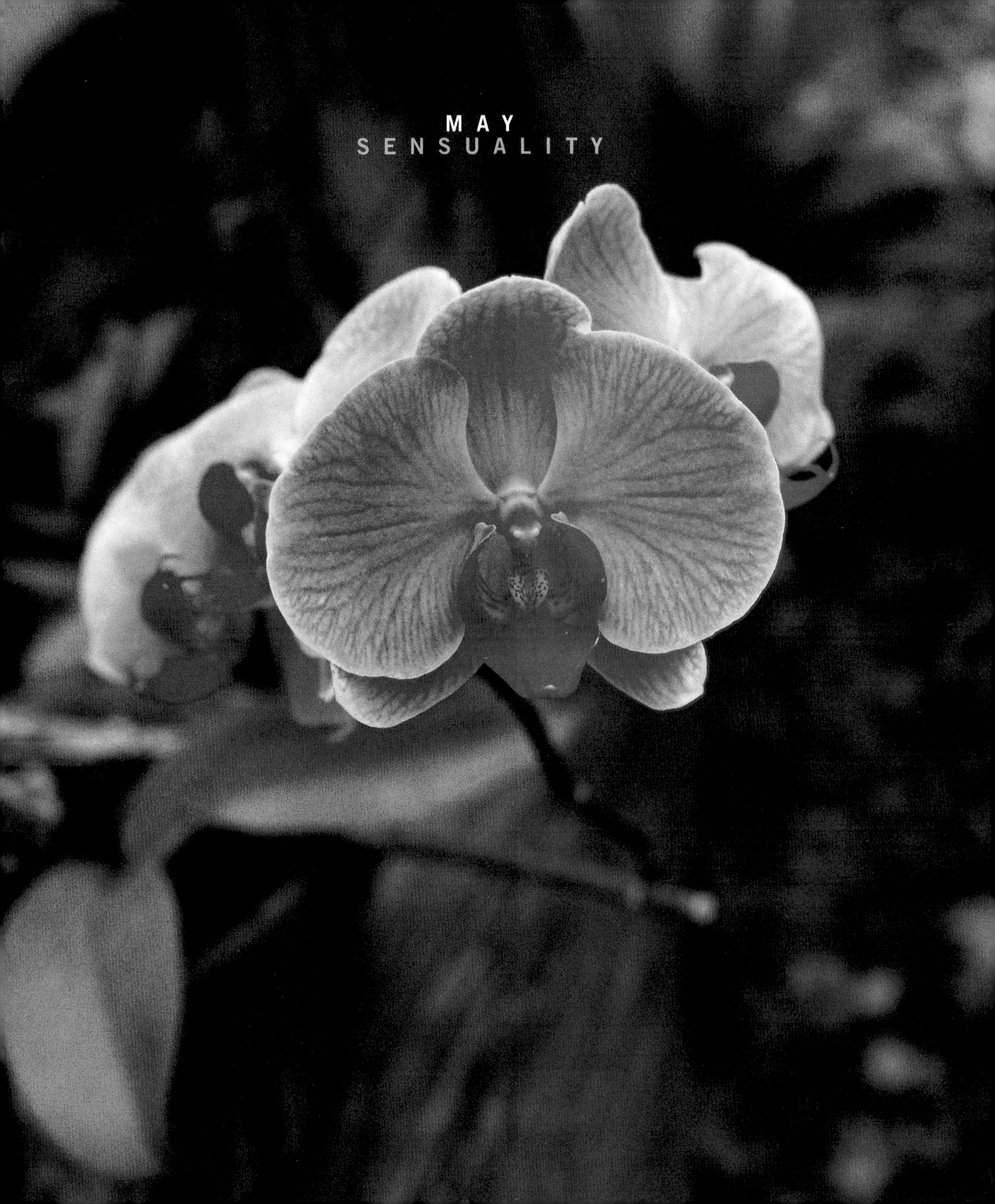

UPDATE YOUR SPRING WARDROBE WITH A FEW NEW ESSENTIAL ACCESSORIES. FOCUS ON SHOES AND HANDBAGS.

1

TAKE A WEEK'S VACATION FROM WATCHING TELEVISION. LISTEN TO MUSIC OR READ INSTEAD.

2

ASK YOUR HAIRSTYLIST TO SHOW YOU TWO OR THREE NEW WAYS TO WEAR YOUR HAIRCUT NEXT TIME YOU GO IN FOR A TRIM.

3

There's no doubt about it—spring is here at last and with it there comes a pleasant sense of anticipation. Soon it will be summer, with its languid days and sultry nights. The pace of life begins to slow as our thoughts turn from pressing deadlines to upcoming vacations and the return to outdoor activities.

As you shed your heavy winter wardrobe, reaching for less structured clothes in gossamer fabrics and cheerful tones, reconnect with the sensual feeling of air on bare skin. Reflect how spring's palette brings a blush to your cheek. Swing a handbag that brings you to life like the flowers and trees around you. Let the breeze toss your hair. You feel sexy, spunky, alive.

Each year I spend part of this month on the French Riviera, working with clients to make their appearance at the world-renowned Cannes Film Festival a smashing success. The contrast between New York's bustle and the languorous heat of the Riviera always highlights for me the inherent sensuality of French women. It's an attitude I'd love to see more women embrace.

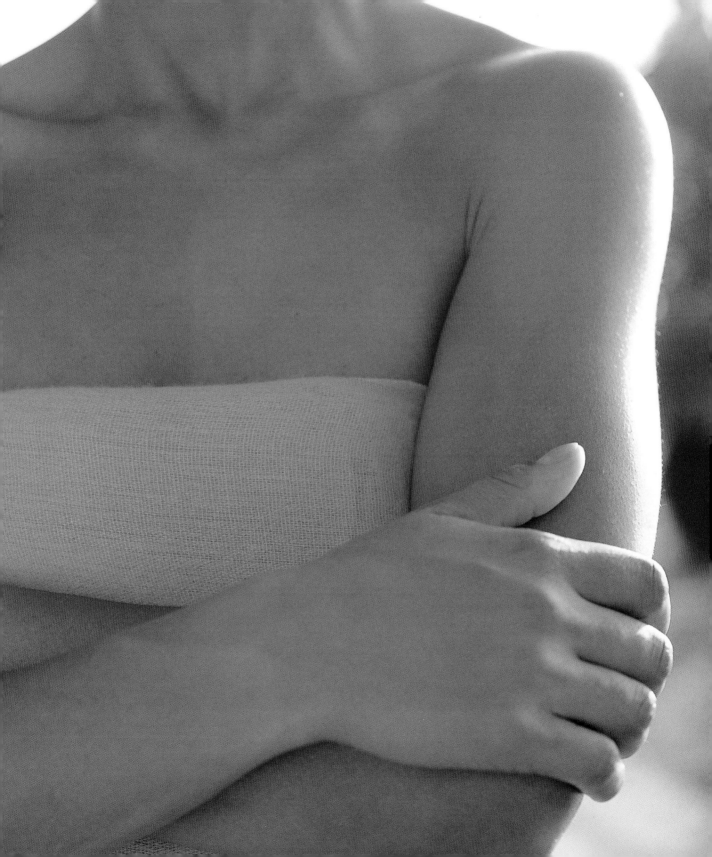

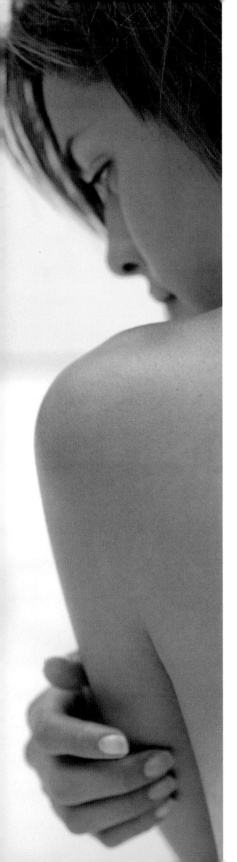

BE SEXY

Being sexy is all in the attitude; it has very little to do with beauty. Nor is sexiness about clothes; you can be sexy in your pajamas if you are in the right mood. And no, sexiness does not come from perfectly applied makeup, the right jewelry, or accessories. So stop asking your mirror who is the sexiest of them all—it's not anything external.

I do think that a particular environment (candles, moonlight, a gorgeous stretch of beach, a fireplace) can make you feel sexier and more attractive. For example, driving a convertible on a beautiful day or walking your dog in the park or on the beach.

Sexiness comes as a result of feeling quietly confident. It's a lighthearted sense of humor that expresses itself in the wit with which you do the most insignificant things: the way you say hello, adjust your sunglasses, hold your bag, cross the street, or get out of your car.

Maybe because I am French, my clients often ask me to define what I call sexy. I don't want to disappoint anyone, but being French doesn't automatically make me an authority on sexiness. As a man who admires women, though, I am glad to offer my humble opinion. For fun, I've made a list of what I find sexy in women. It's totally subjective, so take it with a grain of salt.

AS FAR AS I AM CONCERNED, A WOMAN WHO IS SEXY . . .

* **stands, walks, sits, and moves like a dancer**
* **is playful**
* **carries her bag with ease and elegance**
* **can hold an interesting conversation**
* **hosts any event with charm, grace, and warmth**
* **reads books**
* **wears her hair styled, but not over-styled**
* **has great posture**

* owns a lot of pretty shoes
* holds her fork elegantly
* drinks tea from porcelain cups
* smiles with her eyes
* smells good
* holds her head slightly bent when she listens to me
* wears her hair up with a ribbon to reveal the back of her neck
* makes eye contact across a crowded room

ON THE OTHER HAND, MY LIST OF WHAT'S NOT SEXY INCLUDES:

* dull-looking clothes that hide a woman's sensuality
* a chain and a watch worn together on the same wrist
* bad manners
* makeup on the beach
* clunky shoes
* hair stiff with hairspray
* trying too hard
* over-bleached hair
* fussing in restaurants
* opaque hose for evening
* wearing the wrong clothes for the season
* obvious cleavage
* wrinkled clothes
* piles of gold jewelry
* nails that are too long, artificial, or neglected
* smoking
* talking too loudly
* spending too much time on the phone
* drinking too much
* acting childish

RESOLVE TO FORSWEAR BLACK UNTIL SEPTEMBER—EXCEPT IN THE EVENING.

4

INSTEAD OF SPRAYING ON PERFUME, **A SPLASH OF COLOGNE** IS AN INVIGORATING WAY TO START THE DAY.

5

GO FOR A RUN BEFORE BREAKFAST. **LISTEN TO YOUR FAVORITE CD OF PAVAROTTI**—AND SING ALONG! OXYGENATE YOUR CELLS.

6

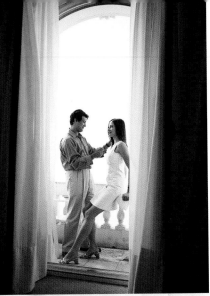

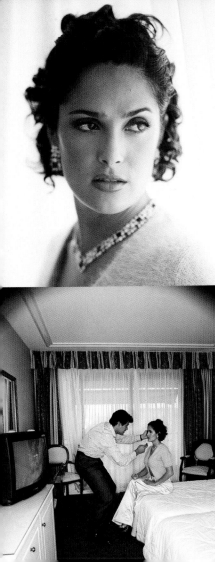

STARLET STYLE

Cannes is a wonderful contrast to Hollywood: Glamour here is much more low-key and relaxed, yet somehow it's so much more sexy. The festival is a series of intimate parties and screenings where people are more comfortable, less on their guard, and always in the mood for a good time.

Because the paparazzi swarm through Cannes with even more ferocity than they invade Hollywood during the Oscars, what they wear and how they look is incredibly important to actresses. But the fact that the event takes place in France adds a touch of joie de vivre: Everyone's just a little giddier, a little more daring, a little sexier than they would be if they were in America. I call the result "starlet style"—pure fun and pure femininity.

Dressing just a tad sexier than you might normally can be energizing as long as you don't overdo it. The line between kittenish and trashy is fine indeed. When in doubt, keep the extra button buttoned, ease up on the eyeliner. The idea is to look sexy, not desperate.

* **WEAR SOMETHING THAT SKIMS THE BODY**, rather than hugs every curve.
* **WEAR SPAGHETTI STRAPS BY ALL MEANS**—they're so sensual. But they don't work with serious cleavage.
* **A STRAPLESS DRESS IS SEXY,** too, but never wear one that's too tight. You'll look like a sausage, no matter how thin you are.
* **HEELS ARE ALMOST ALWAYS SEXIER THAN FLATS,** but if your dress is really sexy, try kitten heels instead of spikes, or even strappy flats. If the dress is more demure, you can be more daring with the shoes.

TOP TO BOTTOM: MIRA SORVINO IS SOPHISTICATED AND GLAMOROUS IN EVERY WAY. SHE KNOWS EXACTLY WHAT TO WEAR— MAKEUP, CLOTHES, ACCESSORIES. SHE IS SIMPLY STUNNING. SALMA HAYEK IS DAZZLING. I LOVE HER NATURAL, FRESH, AND EXOTIC LOOK AND SHE KNOWS HOW TO ACCENTUATE IT GRACIOUSLY. I WORKED WITH BOTH AT THE CANNES FILM FESTIVAL.

* **DETAILS LIKE A LITTLE PEARLED BARRETTE** or a ribbon in the hair show that you thought about your appearance, which is always sexy.
* **DON'T DRESS TOO SERIOUSLY**—evening bags should be original and whimsical to complement what you're wearing.
* **DON'T OVERDO THE ACCESSORIES.** You should wear the accessories, not vice versa.

Starlet style is by no means exclusively for young women. One year at the height of the film festival at Cannes, I was summoned by none other than Elizabeth Taylor. Her Rolls-Royce, complete with police escort, came to whisk me up into the hills, where she received me in her room, a death-defying perch with a panoramic view of the entire Riviera. She had gone blond and wanted a different cut, she explained. "But if you cut my hair wrong, I'll cut your hands off," she added, half-jokingly. Her original cut was a bit too round, too bubble-like for my taste. Making things worse, it was spiky on top. I created a naturally tousled, messy, sex-kitten look, as if she'd just woken up. It was a success. The star of *Cat on a Hot Tin Roof* looked more mischievous and delicious than ever.

SMOLDERING MAKEUP

A sexy dress needs a sexy face to go with it, otherwise you'll be sending a mixed message that says you aren't aware of the impact you're making. A bit of cream blush at the apples of the cheeks makes almost anyone look prettier, younger, and more delectable.

Eyeliner and mascara, judiciously applied, are sexier to me than lots of eye shadow. Focus the liner at the outside corners of the eyes, extending just slightly beyond the top lash line. But beware of smoky eye shadow; too much dark shadow and you'll cross the line from sexy to scary. Lips should be glossy and fairly neutral if you've got a drop-dead-sexy outfit. Red lipstick works only with a more subdued outfit.

SCHEDULE A SERIES OF PEDICURES, ONE EVERY FOUR WEEKS FROM NOW UNTIL SEPTEMBER.

7

OVERCOME YOUR SELF-CONSCIOUSNESS ONCE AND FOR ALL: THINK OF OTHERS, AND SOON YOU'LL FORGET TO THINK ABOUT YOURSELF.

8

No one can make you feel inferior without your consent.
—ELEANOR ROOSEVELT

9

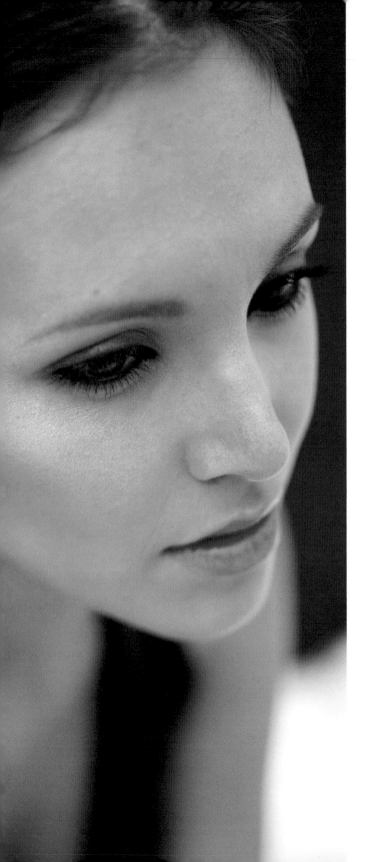

THE SEX KITTEN FACE

An enticing sex kitten face starts with makeup that has a shimmery sheen to it and finishes with more fruity hues on the cheeks and lips—the contrast between the two groups makes the combination sophisticated and fun.

* EYES Choose complementary shadow and pencil in the silvery gray range. The shadow should shimmer and the pencil should be deep. Carefully line close to your lashes all around the eye. With a sponge applicator, apply the shadow over your lid, but not all the way up to the brow. You can also apply a thin stroke of shadow under the eye over the pencil. For an even more intense effect, lightly dampen the sponge before applying another coat of shadow. Blend the pencil and shadow carefully; there should be no obvious lines separating the two colors. Finish with one coat of black mascara.

* LIPS Apply two coats of a brownish peach color to the lips. Once the color completely covers your lips and is even, apply a clear gloss over the color to give your lips a wet, sultry sheen.

* CHEEKS Choose a blush from the peach group (if the color is too pink or red, you'll look more like a china doll). Lightly brush the blush across the apples of your cheeks. The effect should be warm and subtle; you should not be able to distinguish bright spots of peach.

* NAILS Nail polish should be a paler, more shimmery version of the lip color. Look for a color that combines a champagne glow with peachy tones. If you decide to paint your toes, choose a color that's darker and more daring. A rich, metallic wine would complete the look.

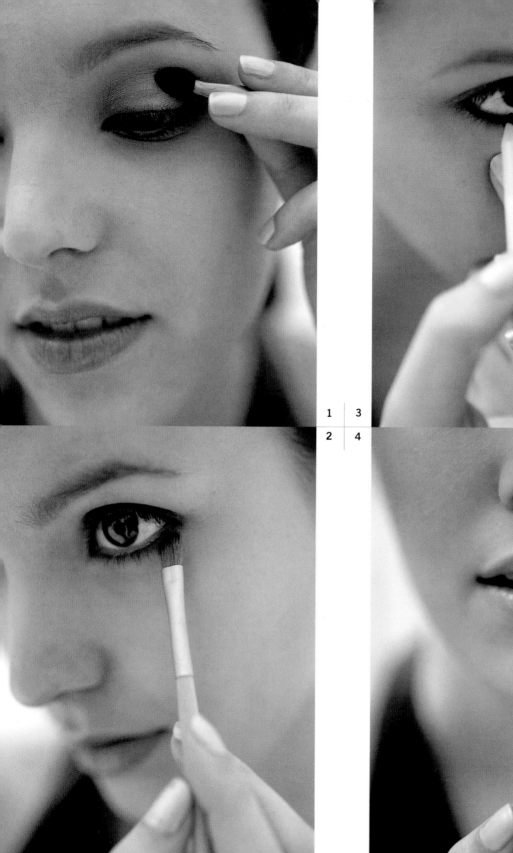

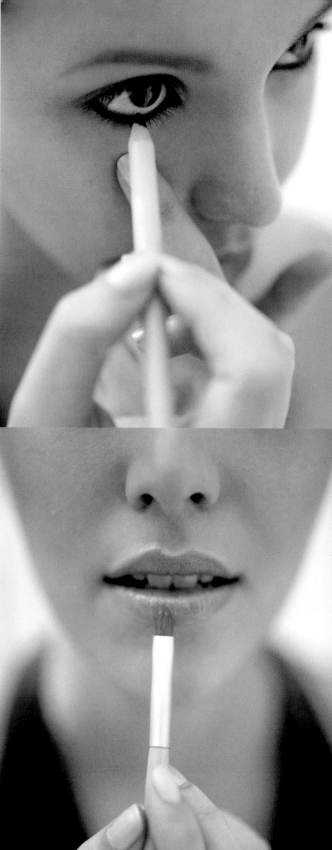

10

MAY MEANS BARER CLOTHING. **EXFOLIATE YOUR SKIN** FROM HEAD TO TOE.

11

BEFORE GOING OUT, **RESHAPE YOUR HAIRSTYLE** WITH A QUICK BLOWOUT. WORK A BIT OF STYLING SPRAY THROUGH YOUR HAIR, HANG YOUR HEAD UPSIDE DOWN, AND BLOW ON LOW HEAT.

12

A CURE FOR INSOMNIA: **TAKE A SALT BATH** WITH LAVENDER ESSENCE BEFORE BEDTIME.

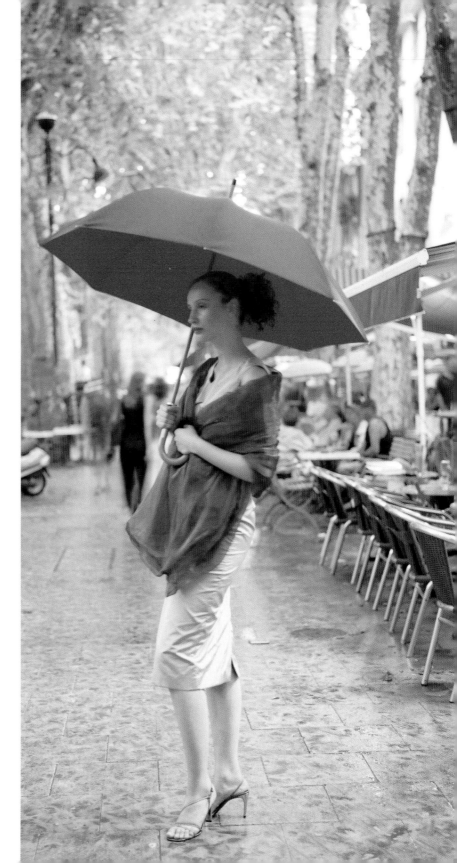

SEXY ACCESSORIES

Let's not confuse sexiness with nakedness! When it comes to looking sensual, less is not always more. Accessories that are only somewhat revealing can make you more alluring than a plunging neckline.

One of the sexiest things a woman can do is create a sense of mystery. Accessories should tease the imagination, suggest the presence of a curve, and draw the attention to a particular spot. Day or night, flirt with a shawl, flash an amusing hair ornament, gesture with your sunglasses—but always in a natural, uncontrived way.

In general, sexy accessories are:

* **small and refined**
* **embellished with touches like feathers, sequins, or beads**
* **playful—with a sense of humor**
* **easy to wear and easy to use**
* **colorful, but not garish**

Wear accessories that fit your personality.

* **IF YOU ARE SHY,** choose a shawl or scarf that kisses your shoulders, allowing just a glimpse of décolletage.
* **IF YOU ARE FLIRTATIOUS,** carry a handbag with small handles, emphasizing the daintiness of your wrists and the movement of your hands.
* **IF YOU ARE OPINIONATED,** wear elegant sunglasses that enhance the intelligence of your face.
* **IF YOU ARE ENERGETIC,** pick a bag with shoulder straps long enough to allow you to move freely.

DON'T WAIT FOR THE LAST MINUTE TO SHOP FOR MOTHER'S DAY.

13

PLACE BUNCHES OF LILACS ALL OVER THE HOUSE, ESPECIALLY RIGHT NEXT TO YOUR BED.

14

The most valuable of arts is the art of living.
—CICERO

15

SOAK YOUR HAIRBRUSHES IN
HOT WATER MIXED WITH A
SPOONFUL OF SHAMPOO FOR
A MINUTE OR TWO, THEN
CLEAN WITH A COMB.

16

DON'T EVER SCOLD YOUR
KIDS—OR ANY CHILD, FOR
THAT MATTER—IN FRONT OF
ADULTS. CALL THEM ASIDE TO
TALK TO THEM.

17

PUT BUTTER ON YOUR TOAST
FROM TIME TO TIME. FAT-
DEFICIENCY MAKES YOUR
HAIR, SKIN, AND NAILS DULL
AND DRY.

18

THE BIG BLOWOUT

What's more sexy than hair that's bouncy, alive, that moves with your body? With your hair sleekly styled, you naturally adopt a more relaxed attitude. You are likely to run your hand through your hair, or push a couple of stray strands off your face with your glasses, or casually re-adjust a hair ornament—all lovely gestures. Beautiful shiny hair, blown out to perfection, is one of the most seductive attributes of a sexy woman.

Blowouts are among the most frequent services we perform at the salon. In the past five years, requests for them have nearly doubled. Some clients have a blowout Monday morning and barely touch their hair for the rest of the week. However, it absolutely depends on your hair texture as to how long a blowout will last. In general, curlier, thicker hair holds a blowout longer, weather permitting: If it's really humid, curly hair is going to lose its style more quickly and revert to its own curly, sometimes frizzy ways.

Women go to the salon for blowouts to get that sleek healthy shine along with a sexy, uplifting bit of volume. They prefer to leave to professionals the task of striking the right balance between using products that enhance the shine of their hair (but can weigh it down, making it flatter), and using volumizers that give it bounce (but can dull its radiance).

It is certainly possible to get the same look at home, if you approach the task with focus. What's most important is to dry the roots first, with hair pulled up, not down, to create bounce and volume, without frizz. I call this overdirecting the roots. Keep these points in mind for the best results:

* **START A BLOWOUT ON DAMP HAIR:** Don't blow out hair that's totally dry. Hair must be humid when you blow-dry it, so that it's elastic and the crinkles can be ironed out.

* **ALWAYS REMEMBER TO POINT THE DRYER DOWN** the shaft of your hair. Going in the other direction disturbs the hair cuticles, and makes it frizzy. So always work downward, pressing the hair with the hot air.

* **THROUGHOUT THE PROCESS,** keep the hair taut between the brush and the nozzle of the dryer. Slide the brush down toward the ends of the hair in concert with the air flow.

* **USE THE NARROW NOZZLE ATTACHMENT** for your blow-dryer so you can direct the flow of air with precision.

* **GRAY HAIR IS DRIER,** meaning coarser and more wiry. To control its texture, apply a mixture of gel and cream before blowing it dry. Only apply gel on wet hair. Apply cream after the blowout, on dry hair.

Once the hair is dry, many stylists finish a blowout with Velcro curlers. Done right, they impart volume at the crown, leave the hair smooth and shiny, and create a sexy flip at the ends. Rollers and curlers can add a sexy energy to a look, without making hair look "curly" per se, but if you're going for that glass-straight look, they are not for you.

Some people like hot rollers, which I don't generally recommend. When you're doing your own hair in front of a mirror, I think it's just a recipe for trouble. If you're good at it, fine. Just remember to do it before you put in any finishing cream, and don't leave the rollers in too long, they'll fry your hair. Always brush your hair out with a flat brush after you've taken out the curlers.

I don't like the fried, artificial look that curling irons leave on hair, except for the rare special occasion (see page 286). For everyday, do any curling you need to do while you're drying the hair, with a round brush.

SELECTING THE PERFECT BRUSH

A well-made, high-quality hairbrush is an essential tool for creating salon-perfect hair at home. But it's equally important to choose the right brush for your hair in order to get the desired results.

* **FOR SHORT HAIRSTYLES:** Use a brush with a small, perferated metal body when blow-drying.

* **FOR CHIN- TO SHOULDER-LENGTH HAIRSTYLES:** Blow-dry using a round, medium-size brush with natural bristles.

* **TO STRAIGHTEN LONG HAIR:** Use a large, flat brush with natural bristles.

* **FOR NATURALLY STRAIGHT HAIR:** Use a flat brush. Don't bother with a blow-dryer, though. To add volume and shine, simply brush your hair three to four times a day in all directions.

THE ULTIMATE STEP-BY-STEP BLOWOUT

To get salon-perfect results at home, follow the same steps your stylist does:

✳ FIRST, FLIP YOUR HEAD OVER and dry your hair upside down until it's 70 percent dry, with little regard for how it looks.

✳ FLIP YOUR HAIR BACK UP, and dry the roots.

✳ USING A FLAT BRUSH, take a section of hair and overdirect the roots, that is, use the brush to pull the hair against its natural direction and direct the air flow *down* the hair shaft. Dry, dry, dry. Spray volumizer on the roots.

✳ AFTER YOU'VE SPRITZED IN THE VOLUMIZER, take a round brush and bend the hair at the roots. Overdirect the roots, then pull the brush through to the ends. Don't turn the brush; it rubs your hair in the wrong way and creates frizz.

✳ WHEN YOUR HAIR IS COMPLETELY DRY, rub a little finishing cream on your fingers and rake them through your hair (mostly at the ends) to add a little texture and make it less puffy. Be careful; too much cream will make hair limp and greasy-looking.

✳ WITH LONG HAIR, use a round brush, going from the roots to the ends, without turning the brush (which makes your arm and wrist tired for no good reason). Work to get a bend in the roots right up at the top for volume and movement, then just slide the brush down, with the dryer following (always pointed down), to the end, which should also get just a little bend, a little flip.

✳ FOR SHORT HAIR, always use a flat brush, and really play with it as you dry in different directions, even against the part. As it gets dry, it will fall into place, but remain slightly tousled, which is always sexy.

✳ IF YOU WANT TO GET EXTRA VOLUME, dry your roots first. Lift your hair at a 60 degree angle, place your brush against the scalp, and lay your hair over it. Point your blow-dryer at the roots and dry. Next, dry the tip of your hair with the dryer pointing downward.

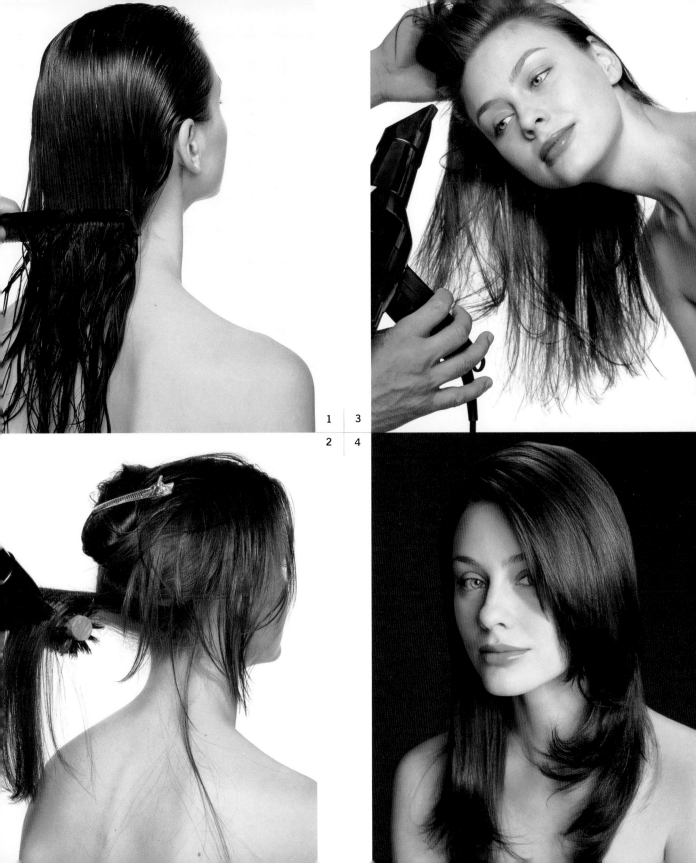

1 | 3
2 | 4

STYLING PRODUCTS

Almost every client I've ever had has questions about the incredible range of creams, mousses, sprays, gels, pomades, and texturizers that are out there, all promising to make hair more beautiful, often in similar-sounding ways.

All styling products change your hair's texture in some way: They'll give it more volume, or they'll make it softer, more pliable. They'll make it stiffer, so it stays in one place, or they can make it stickier, so it holds together better and is less frizzy. The right texture can make your hair look healthier; it can even highlight color in a way that your natural texture might not. It can make your hair easier to work with or impossible to work with. So knowing which product does what—a nearly impossible task if the product labels are all you have to go on—is critical.

HAIR SPRAY AND VOLUMIZING SPRAY Volumizing spray adds fullness, especially to long, fine hair. Lift the hair up and spritz on at the roots before styling as usual.

Do spray through the hair, not just on top. Or spray your brush with hair spray and brush through. This gives great support and hold without weighing down the hair. You'll get a better, softer look, too.

MOUSSE Mousse is absolutely wonderful for fine hair, because it beefs up the hair's texture and gives it a bit of structure, so it will stay where you put it— the biggest problem for women with fine hair. But here's the caveat: I really only use it in short hair. With long hair, the texture is too much, and it sticks hair together in clumps and leaves it with a flat finish. The movement of a short haircut will mask all of that, including the finish, and the mousse will give short hair really long-lasting volume and shape.

So use mousse only if you've got short and fine hair.

GEL Use gel to give both volume and support to any straight hairstyle, short or long, but use it only at the roots. Working in gel beyond the roots defeats its purpose: It's so heavy that anywhere else on the hair, gravity does its work and pulls the hair down, so it ends up flatter than when you started.

Don't use gel at all if you've got curly hair. It makes it crunchy and dull-looking; try a finishing cream instead.

FINISHING CREAMS, POMADES, AND OILS Finishing creams are only for the ends of the hair, to define them a bit, and make hair shinier and healthy-looking. They work with almost any hairstyle, on curly or straight hair, but they must always be used very sparingly. They can make your hair look greasy very easily, if you use even a bit too much.

Pomades, waxes, and hair oils are generally more intense than creams, you need even less of them. And only very frizzy, rough-textured hair needs something like an oil at all.

Always take a little bit of the cream (or the pomade or oil) and rub it between your hands until it's very well distributed across them; then run just your fingers through the ends of your hair. If you need more, repeat the process.

STRAIGHTENING BALM This is a wonderful product that enables those with very curly hair to achieve the look of straight hair. It should be worked into towel-dried hair then combed through. The hair can be left to air dry for a softly waxy style, or blown dry with a round brush to straighten the hair completely.

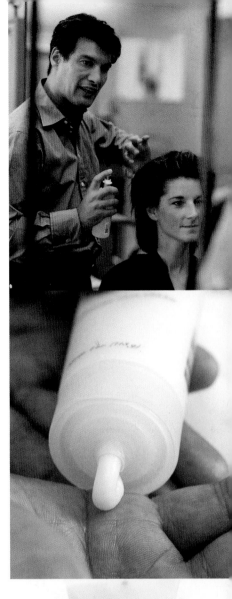

25 PRACTICE POSING FOR PHOTOGRAPHS IN FRONT OF A MIRROR. LOOK AT YOUR SMILE. DO YOUR EYES TWINKLE?

26 **STAY LIMBER BY WALKING** AROUND THE ROOM EVERY HOUR. INVEST IN A CORDLESS TELEPHONE TO PACE WHILE YOU TALK.

27 CALL YOUR FLORIST OR AN ON-LINE SERVICE AND **SEND SOMEONE FLOWERS** JUST FOR THE FUN OF IT.

LOOKING GREAT
IN PHOTOGRAPHS

Learning to look at yourself in photographs is as tricky as learning to look at yourself in mirrors. Bad snapshots taken by well-meaning relatives can damage your self-confidence more than the most critical self-scrutiny.

Like most people, I hate posing for photographs. But, over the years, watching many of my famous clients pose over and over for paparazzi shots (not to mention official portraits, and the thousands of model shoots I've been on), I've picked up a few things.

MAKEUP

* **USE AS LITTLE FOUNDATION** and powder as you can when having a picture taken; you want your skin as natural-looking as possible. Heavy eye makeup or very stiff hair, likewise, looks so unnatural.

* **BLACK-AND-WHITE PHOTOGRAPHY** is especially crisp, making any cosmetics you wear more noticeable. Your makeup should be defined but natural, perhaps just a bit of mascara, a touch of blush, a bit of liner or shadow, but never both. Choose a completely neutral lipstick, or even just a gloss: Dark lipstick looks just awful in black-and-white pictures.

* **COLOR PICTURES ARE A LITTLE MORE FORGIVING.** Pay special attention to your eyes, brows, and lips: Define them; make sure they stand out (though you don't want the color of your makeup to stand out). A little eyeliner, a darker lip, and a bit of brow pencil will highlight your face without looking overly made-up.

RIGHT: PROFESSIONAL MODELS KNOW HOW TO ROMANCE THE CAMERA. A WARM SMILE ALWAYS WORKS.

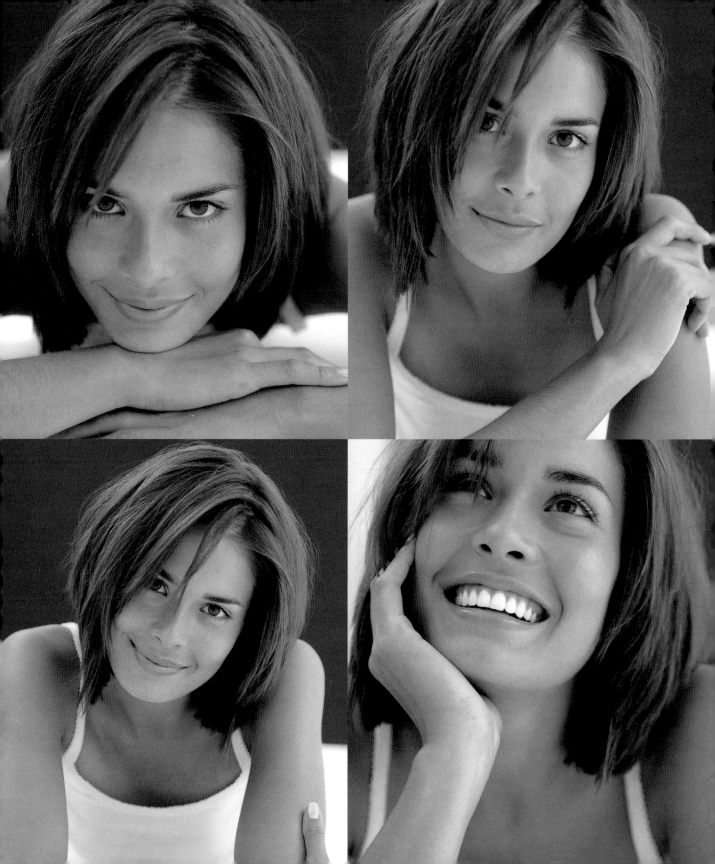

28 START A NEW EXERCISE
REGIMEN THAT ENCOURAGES
YOU TO SPEND AS MUCH TIME
AS POSSIBLE OUTSIDE.

29 DRINK MORE WATER,
PREFERABLY WITHOUT
BUBBLES. ALMOST EVERYONE
COULD DRINK A LITTLE MORE.

30 SURPRISE YOUR PARENTS
WITH THEATER TICKETS.

31 MAKE YOUR HAIR SHINE BY
RINSING IT WITH FRESH
LEMON JUICE AND WATER.

HAIR

* **HAIR FOR BOTH COLOR AND BLACK-AND-WHITE PICTURES** should be together, styled but not overdone, shiny and healthy-looking. Black-and-white film plays up hair's texture, so make sure it is lustrous.
* **IF YOU KNOW THAT YOU ARE GOING TO BE PHOTOGRAPHED** for a portrait, have a haircut a week before, to give your hair time to settle.
* **MANY PEOPLE BRUSH THEIR HAIR JUST BEFORE** taking a picture. This can cause a bit of frizz, so take along a bit of finishing cream.

CLOTHES

* **THE RIGHT CLOTHES FOR ANY PORTRAIT** are the simplest. Fussy patterns or over-engineered designs take the focus away from you. Trendy clothes will make the photo look dated in a few years.
* **COLORS THAT FLATTER YOU OFF-CAMERA** will usually work well on film, too. Blue—practically any shade of it—looks fantastic on almost everyone, and it looks just as good in black-and-white as in color film.
* **SHOULD YOU EVER HAVE TO APPEAR ON TELEVISION,** always wear a solid primary pastel color that complements your skin tone. Even on the worst-quality video, it holds up and looks cool and calm.

LIGHT

* **HOW YOU'RE GOING TO LOOK IN A PHOTOGRAPH** depends first and foremost on the available light. The most flattering light to be photographed in is what photographers call "open shade": a bright, sunny day and both you and the photographer are in full shade. A close second is at sunset.
* **IT SHOULD GO WITHOUT SAYING** that fluorescent light is the least flattering. Midday sun and flashbulb-light are not much better. Try to avoid them.

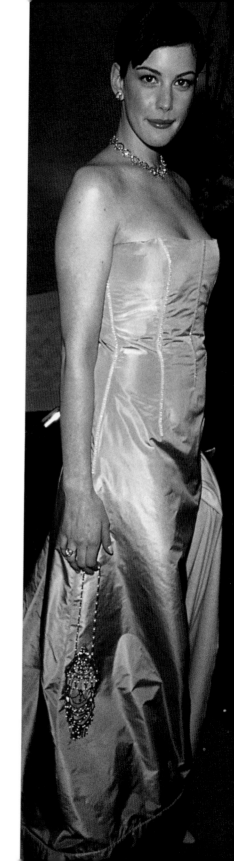

* **STUDIO LIGHTING DEPENDS ENTIRELY ON THE LIGHTING TALENTS** of the photographer. If you're having a portrait taken, select someone who's lighting and end photographs you've seen and liked.

BACKGROUND

* **CHOOSE TO BE PHOTOGRAPHED** in front of a plain background. Don't stand in front of a painting or against garish wallpaper.
* **FOR CANDID TRAVEL PICTURES,** a quiet landscape makes the best backdrop. Crowded street scenes can throw weird shadows across your face, and looming landmarks can distort the proportions of the setting.
* **IN A STUDIO,** background music will help you relax and look upbeat.
* **DON'T STAND IN FRONT OF GREEN PLANTS OR HEDGES.**

POSTURE

* **THE MAIN POINT IS THE HARDEST:** Look natural and relaxed. Forget the camera. Easier said than done, but if you can do it, you'll look great.
* **SMILE.** It takes years off your face.
* **KEEP YOUR CHIN TILTED SLIGHTLY UPWARD.**
* **SWALLOW.** It makes your posture better, and it makes your neck look longer and more graceful.
* **A VERY FAMOUS MODEL** who's often shot in tiny bikinis once told me that she pushes her shoulders forward, to minimize her bottom half.
* **FOR LONG PHOTO SESSIONS,** keep a glass of water or champagne, whatever pleases you, close by.
* **LAST BUT NOT LEAST:** Have the photographer shoot lots of film, always. He's bound to catch you looking sexy, natural, and friendly.

RIGHT: LIV TYLER'S 1999 OSCAR LOOK WAS EFFORTLESSLY ELEGANT; I SLICKED HER HAIR BACK AND TIED IT WITH A LEATHER STRING FROM HER MANOLO BLAHNIKS.

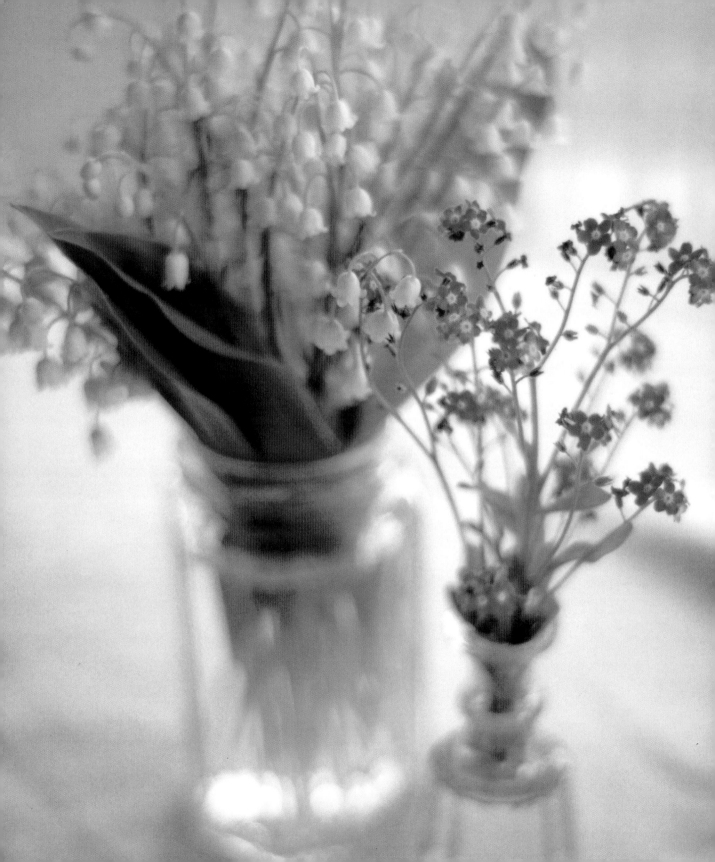

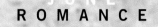

JUNE
ROMANCE

1 HAVE YOUR WINTER COATS AND SUITS VACUUM-PACKED AT THE DRY CLEANERS AND STORE THEM UNTIL YOU NEED THEM.

2 **DON'T SCUFF YOUR HIGH HEELS.** KEEP DRIVING SHOES IN THE CAR, AS WELL AS GREAT MUSIC, TISSUES, AND WATER.

3 **JUNE IS THE BEST MONTH FOR ROSES.** BUY A CRYSTAL VASE TALL ENOUGH FOR THE LONG-STEMMED BEAUTIES.

Why is it that the longer the days and the shorter the nights, the more likely we are to fall in love? Beware of the month of June. The summer solstice is conducive to infatuation. June weddings are the most romantic. And with everyone around you exchanging vows and tying the knot, how can you not be in an amorous mood?

If you develop an unexpected summer crush on a less-than-perfect mate, don't fight it. Opposites attract, and that's that. I have a friend who is generous, friendly, laid-back, and never on edge. In contrast, his wife is high-strung and brittle. Yet they are patient toward each other, still in love after many years together. How can this be, his friends wonder. Live and learn. When I see them, I can't help but admire their style as a couple. Sincere kindness between a man and a woman is a real class act.

RIGHT: THE SENSE OF SMELL IS A DOOR TO SWEET MEMORIES AND ROMANCE.

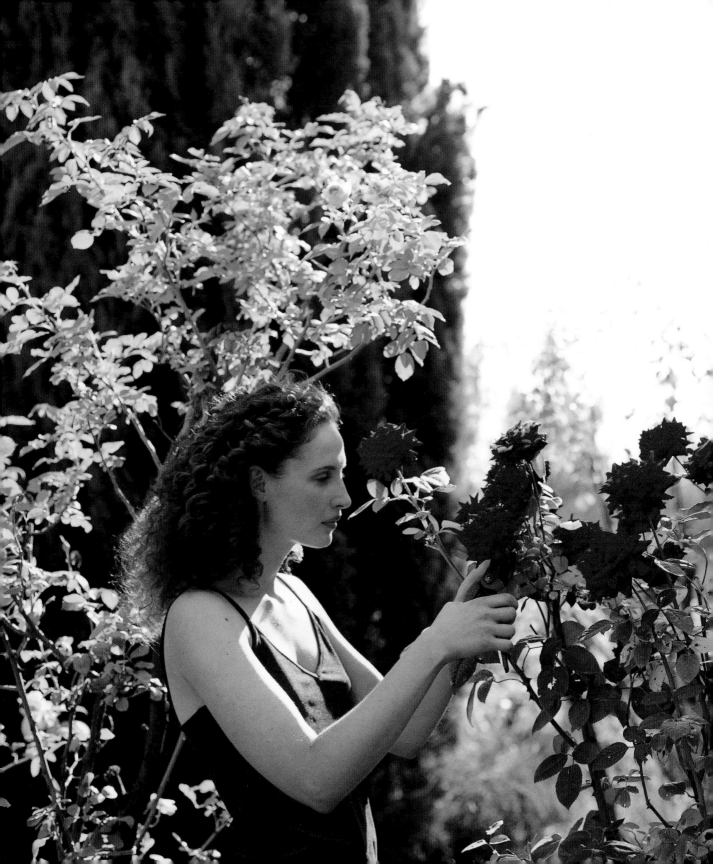

4   **ORDER YOUR FATHER A GIFT CERTIFICATE** FOR A MASSAGE FOR FATHER'S DAY.

5   **GO HIKING.** STANDING ON TOP OF A MOUNTAIN GIVES YOU A NEW PERSPECTIVE ON LIFE.

6   IF YOUR HAIR IS LIGHT, ASK YOUR HAIR COLORIST TO **ADD EXTRA HIGHLIGHTS** FOR THE SUMMER.

THE RULES OF ROMANCE

I have been in and out of the single scene longer than I care to admit, and each time I find myself dating again, I realize how important kindness is in the game of love. If I had one piece of advice to give anyone who is starting in a relationship, I would say, "Learn to listen." Being attentive and giving the other the opportunity to talk is the most tender expression of love.

The rules of courtship have evolved (for the better) but certain universals never change. First and foremost, be yourself. Then:

* **Turn off your cell phone when on a date.**
* **Don't go out of your way to be controversial.**
* **When you talk, don't just fill the hole in conversation; add something of substance.**
* **Don't lie about your accomplishments.**
* **Don't pretend to be cool.**
* **Compliment your date on his style; it shows that you have good taste.**
* **Wear the same fragrance every time: leave your mark with a scented signature.**
* **After a fight, acknowledge how silly you were: send flowers and apologize in a nice way—particularly if you were right.**

Because of my profession, I talk to a lot of women. And I have never met a female client who didn't have something unique to teach me. There is never a dull moment in my salons. I am not shy about letting my male friends know how lucky I consider myself for working with so many members of the opposite sex.

RIGHT: ABOVE ALL, BE WITH SOMEONE WHO MAKES YOU SMILE.

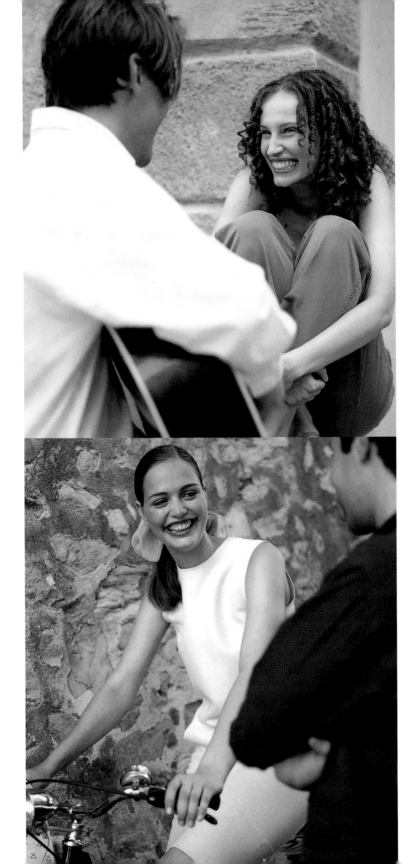

FOR WOMEN ONLY...

* Be his friend first, his girlfriend second.

* Dress for yourself; don't change your style.

* Don't compete with him: Let him open the door for you if he offers.

* Be considerate: Offer to lend him an umbrella if it rains, or a sweater if it's cold.

* Don't do too much to please him, it's a sure sign that you are desperate. When he comes to your house, offer him a drink, but don't serve him. Let him open the bottle and pour.

FOR MEN ONLY...

* Wait patiently while she gets ready.

* Be a gentleman: Open doors and carry packages.

* Compliment her hair, but not her figure.

* If she asks you to do something, do it at once. Don't wait until it's convenient for you.

7

OVERTIP FOR NO SPECIAL REASON. ALWAYS TIP, EVEN IF YOU'RE A GUEST.

8

The days that make us happy make us wise.

—JOHN MASEFIELD

9

BUY FRESH MINT AND FREEZE IN ICE CUBES FOR SUMMER DRINKS.

WEDDINGS
GETTING MARRIED IN STYLE

When a man and a woman decide to get married, they usually have no idea how complicated it is to organize a wedding. Ignorance is bliss. Soon enough they discover that the process can be grueling, and far from romantic. In my opinion, too much time, money, and effort is wasted on details that don't necessarily reflect the spirit of the two people involved. The most important thing about a wedding is to preserve its gaiety.

I hear a great deal about weddings all year long. I've spent countless hours preparing for them, in one way or another: Planning with a woman how she can look and feel more beautiful than she's ever been. Styling entire bridal parties. Giving advice to a nervous but stylish mother-of-the-bride.

How formal you make a wedding depends entirely on your personality and your style, but also on the location, the time of day, and the season. I remember, for instance, going to a wedding in Los Angeles in a tiny church on a hill. What was most memorable about the event was a detail most people would have overlooked: The ceremony took place in the late afternoon, just before sunset, when the light was at its most beautiful.

When I got married, like so many people, I didn't take the time to visualize exactly what my mood would be given the circumstances. Because the wedding was to take place on St. Barthélemy, I assumed that I should wear a wonderful white summer suit, the best I could find, to match the smart, short, raw-silk dress that Catherine, my wife-to-be, had bought for the occasion. At the last minute, I came to my senses and realized that my *Saturday Night Fever* suit would be too "done" for the setting. I went to a local shop and got a pair of classic white Bermuda shorts and a beautiful navy polo shirt in the finest cotton, an outfit much more suited to the weather of the island. After lunch that day, we set sail on a catamaran, where the ceremony took place. Minutes after I kissed the bride my friends threw me into the ocean, and everyone ended up jumping in after me in a joyous, spur-of-the-moment gesture.

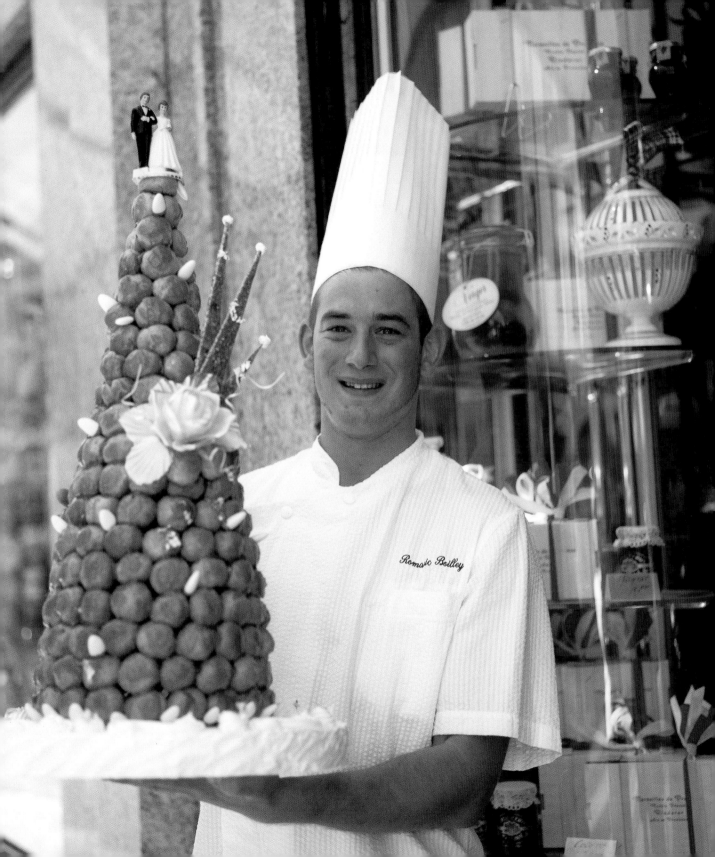

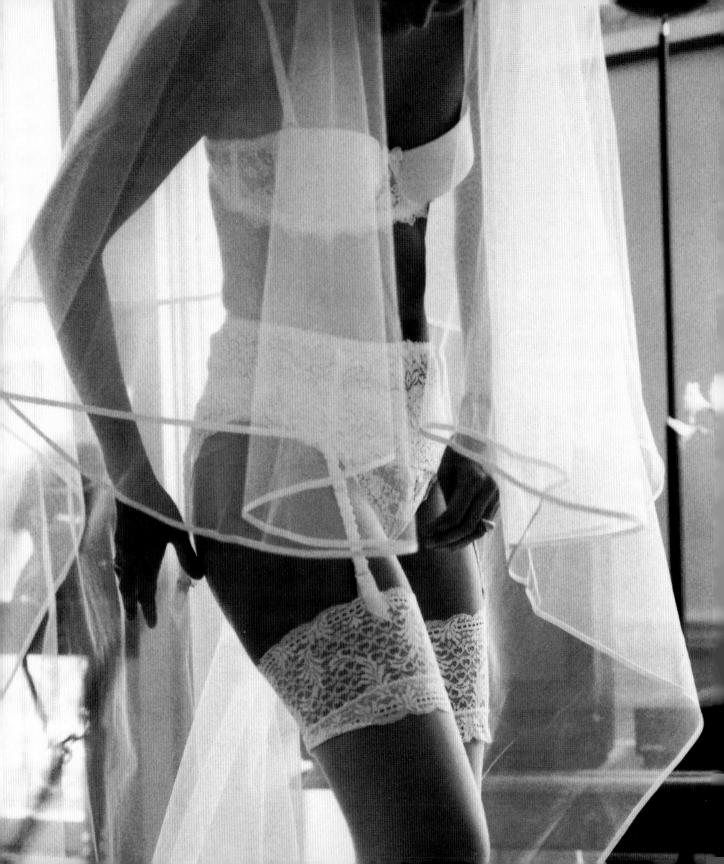

BRIDAL STYLE

PICKING A DRESS My clients bring their wedding dresses to the salon so I can get an idea of what's going to work in terms of hair, makeup, and accessories. Getting married is the best time to make a big deal out of the smallest things . . . in a good way. The right dress makes the bride feel beautiful—it's as simple as that. There are, however, a few caveats:

* **YOU'RE NOT OUT TO SEDUCE ANYONE AT A WEDDING** (presumably, in some capacity, that has been accomplished), so don't dress that way.
* **ON THE OTHER HAND,** avoid fabrics or styles that hide your body completely. I'm thinking, say, of layers and layers of crinoline combined with long, puffed sleeves, a high neck, buttons, lace, embroidery, and cutwork all piled into one design; Victorian is never flattering.
* **NEVER BUY THE FIRST THING YOU TRY ON** until you've seen many other options.
* **EVEN IF YOU PLAN TO HAVE YOUR DRESS CUSTOM-MADE,** try on some ready-to-wear dresses to get an idea of what works for you and what doesn't.
* **HAVE FUN.** Bring your mother or your girlfriends. If all goes according to plan, you'll only get to do this once in your life.

HAIR Hair for weddings is tricky. You want to look styled, groomed, but you don't want anything that isn't absolutely, completely you. In other words, you need to look as though you've made an effort, but haven't gone over the top. Making matters worse, your hairstyle must last all day, and it must look natural despite the veils, hats, and other accoutrements of a wedding. A bride's hair, above all, should be shiny, soft, and free.

* **IF YOU CAN, CONSULT YOUR HAIRDRESSER SIX MONTHS IN ADVANCE.** Discuss whether or not you want to grow your hair for the occasion. Do you want to look casual or dressy?

CALL YOUR PARENTS, JUST TO SEE HOW THEY'RE DOING. 10

MOVE YOUR TIRED AND DROOPY HOUSEPLANTS INTO THE GARDEN TO REJUVENATE THEM. 11

GET A GOOD SUNSCREEN, OR EVEN BETTER, ONE OF THE LATEST SEE-THROUGH SUN BLOCKS. 12

THROW A LITTLE DINNER PARTY FOR FRIENDS WHO GOT MARRIED RECENTLY, SO THEY CAN SHOW THEIR LOVE FOR EACH OTHER IN A MORE RELAXED SETTING.

13

HAVE A NATURAL HEALING REIKU MASSAGE TO REVITALIZE BOTH BODY AND SOUL.

14

TAKE UP A NEW SUMMER ACTIVITY. TRY GARDENING OR PAINTING OR ANYTHING YOU CAN DO OUTDOORS.

15

* **PLAN TO TRY SEVERAL STYLES** with your hairdresser in the months leading up to your wedding. Bring your dress (or a Polaroid of it) to the salon, along with the veil and maybe even the jewelry you plan to wear. Be patient, take the time to experiment with a few different ideas.

* **DON'T CUT OR COLOR YOUR HAIR AT THE LAST MINUTE**—even with the most experienced stylist, accidents do happen. Leave enough time to fix anything that might potentially go wrong. Color, especially, can look a little too opaque at first. Only after you wash it a few times does it become a little more transparent and natural.

* **KEEP IN MIND** that getting used to your new look two to three weeks before the event will help you feel more relaxed at the altar.

* **REMEMBER THAT SQUEAKY-CLEAN HAIR** has a harder time holding a style. On your wedding day, after washing it, your stylist will need to use a little more gel or finishing cream than usual to "dirty" it a bit, to give it more hold and texture.

* **WITH SHORT HAIR,** think about accentuating texture. Bring out different "pieces" of hair to emphasize its color.

* **WITH MID-LENGTH HAIR,** a bob tucked very cleanly behind the ears is very becoming, particularly when held in place with a white satin ribbon or a little barrette, perhaps with freshwater pearls.

* **WITH LONG HAIR,** opt for a loose chignon, with part of the hair falling down around the shoulders, maybe with a soft wave. To get it right, start with a set in large rollers, nothing too fancy, and then have some pieces up in the chignon, some falling down.

* **A HEADDRESS** is something to consider as well. But keep in mind that veils and head ornaments are most appropriate for very young brides.

RIGHT: IF YOU USUALLY WEAR YOUR HAIR DOWN, DON'T AUTOMATICALLY CHOOSE AN UPDO FOR YOUR WEDDING. SOFT ROMANTIC CURLS MAKE THIS STRAIGHT HAIR POLISHED AND PRETTY.

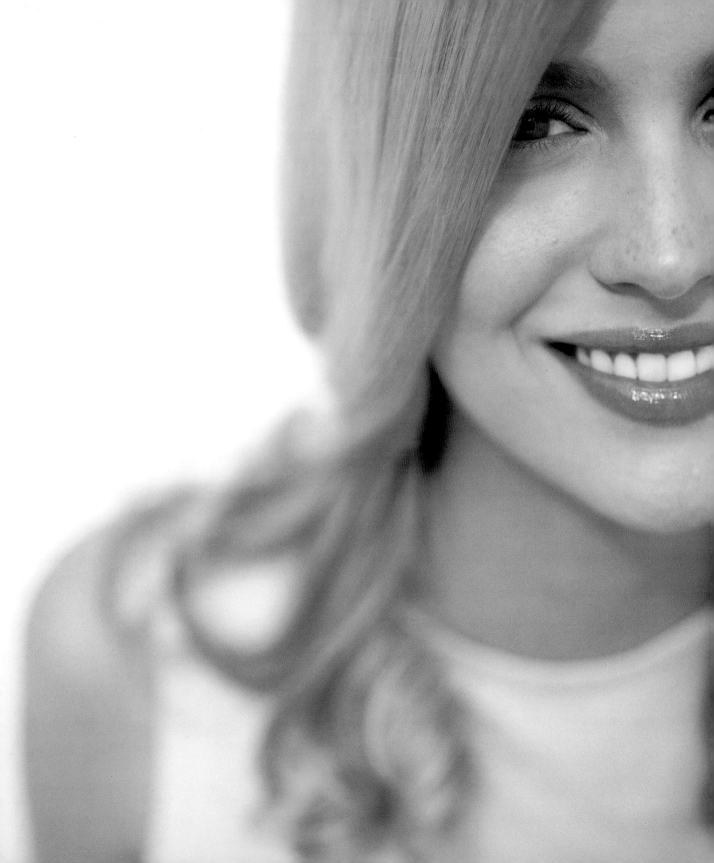

EASE A HANGOVER BY
SOAKING IN A TUB OF HOT
16 WATER SCENTED WITH
FENNEL, JUNIPER, AND
ROSEMARY OILS.

**INVEST IN A GREAT PAIR OF
SANDALS.** AND NEVER WEAR
17 STOCKINGS WITH SANDALS. IT
JUST DOESN'T WORK.

**CHOOSE SUNGLASSES WITH
COLORED LENSES**; IT WILL
18 KEEP YOU IN A HAPPY MOOD
ALL SUMMER.

MAKEUP Some makeup artists encourage brides to wear more makeup than they normally would, reasoning that people in the audience won't be able to see their features well enough. I couldn't disagree more—this is not a stage production! You'll be seeing almost everyone face to face at some point during the event, and you'll be photographed at close range. If the wedding is during the day, you'll be in daylight, which is the most unforgiving light for makeup—meaning people will see almost every bit of it on your face. Instead concentrate your efforts on perfecting your skin: Careful concealer, foundation, powder. Keep eyes as natural as possible, and lips as simple as possible. Blush should be no more or less than you'd wear on a night out to a restaurant. And perhaps it goes without saying, but your mascara definitely needs to be waterproof.

Create a little touch-up kit. When you're about to pose for photographs, for instance, you'll need extra powder to keep from looking shiny in the pictures. Keep a little compact with you or have one of your bridesmaids carry it. Ditto for your sheer, natural-looking lipstick, and some concealer.

If you're having an evening wedding, the light will be more forgiving, and you can afford to wear a little more makeup. But again, don't go overboard. Keep the focus on your personality. Either way, practice the look a few times, and at least once if you're using a makeup artist. Make sure it's right for you, that you feel comfortable, natural, and utterly yourself. Have you ever heard someone say, "Too bad the bride didn't wear more makeup"?

NAILS Go short. Long nails on a bride are just wrong. For evening, colors like a deep, classic red are fine, otherwise, I'd go with very pale pink or clear. If you must have wild polish, put it on your toes.

RIGHT: A SLICK OF SHEER, NATURAL-TONED LIP GLOSS AND A
SHEER PASTEL EYE SHADOW (PLUS WATERPROOF MASCARA!)
MAKE A PERFECT BRIDAL LOOK.

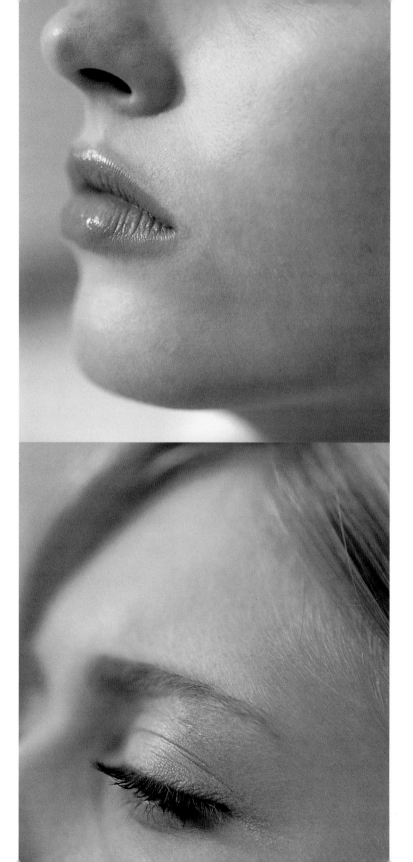

BUYING A
WEDDING GIFT

Of course, most people are registered with a store, and it's fine to choose something from their list, but I think wedding gifts should be more personal. Instead of the obligatory set of candlesticks, consider the following:

✳ AN OBJECT REMINISCENT of a joke or special moment you once shared.

✳ CARDS ENGRAVED with the couple's new address.

✳ A DONATION to their favorite charity.

✳ A BOXED SET of CDs of an artist they love.

✳ A GORGEOUS ENCYCLOPEDIA.

✳ TOPIARIES in shapes that might make them laugh.

HOW TO MAKE A MEMORABLE TOAST

A memorable toast always involves a fabulous anecdote, with heartfelt emotions expressed as plainly as possible. The best toast makes everyone laugh and cry.

* Think of giving a toast as paying tribute to a loved one.

* Humor is often the best way to illuminate what's wonderful about a person, and everyone loves to laugh. But make sure your jokes are PG-rated, even if there are no children present.

* Practice what you plan to say.

* Stay focused on a few key points. Aim to express what it is you love most about the person.

* Short can indeed be the sweetest, especially if you're nervous.

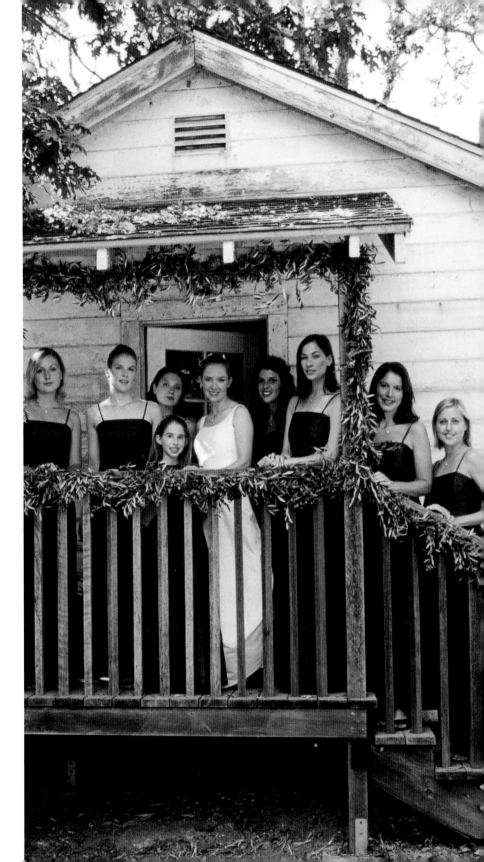

JEWELRY More than any other day of your life, your wedding celebrates who you are, not your accessories, your makeup, or your nails. So keep your jewelry subtle, small, and sentimental—something that has meaning for you. Almost any stone is fine for a wedding, so long as it's tiny.

SHOES Especially if you're wearing a long dress, be particular about comfort. You're going to be standing for a very, very long time. If you're comfortable with literally kicking up (and off) your heels once the reception gets going, go for gorgeous, high, strappy sandals.

GROOMSMEN AND BRIDESMAIDS

If you can afford it, have hair and makeup people, even manicurists and pedicurists, for the bridal party on the morning of the wedding. It helps keep everyone cheerful. The looks should be planned in advance with the stylists, during a consultation, so there are no surprises and everyone can just relax. Even if you can't afford hiring a couple of stylists (though this is money well spent), just arrange for one person you trust to help everyone as they're getting ready. A little advice can go a long way. Make this moment a festive occasion. And have the photographer stop by for a few candid shots.

The fashion industry, for whatever reason, has forsaken the poor bridesmaid. I know of no other category of dresses so universally unflattering. A few ideas: Shop for the dress in a regular store, or with a designer you love. Or, choose a fabric instead of a dress, then let your bridesmaids determine, individually, how their own dresses should be designed. The look is still somewhat cohesive, because of the fabric, and it's charming, because it allows their personalities to shine through.

Whenever possible, include children in the ceremony. For my second wedding, to Elizabeth Shiell, our son Alexandre was my best man. When he saw our two rings on the little pillow, he asked: "Where is my ring?" His remark was the high point of the ceremony.

SHOP FOR CLOTHES AFTER A PLEASANT LUNCH, WHEN YOU FEEL RELAXED. IF YOU ARE TENSE, YOU WILL NEVER BE SATISFIED WITH WHAT YOU FIND.

19

TREAT A FRIEND TO A VISIT TO THE COSMETICS COUNTER AND HELP HER UPDATE HER LOOK. IT'S MORE FUN THAN BUYING SOMETHING FOR YOURSELF.

20

CELEBRATE THE SUMMER SOLSTICE BY TAKING A SWIM UNDER THE STARS.

21

CHERRIES ARE IN SEASON:
MAKE A QUICK CLAFOUTI BY
COMBINING 1 CUP OF SOUR
CREAM, 1 CUP RICOTTA
CHEESE, ½ CUP FLOUR,
3 TABLESPOONS SUGAR, AND
2 EGGS. STIR AND POUR INTO
A PYREX PIE DISH. ADD 2 CUPS
OF PITTED CHERRIES. BAKE
AT 350°F FOR 45 MINUTES.
SPRINKLE SUGAR ON TOP.

22

**PUSH YOUR CUTICLES BACK
WITH CREAM** AFTER WASHING
YOUR HANDS.

23

AFTER A SHAMPOO, **GIVE
YOUR HAIR AN INSTANT WAVE**
BY TWISTING IT ON TOP OF
YOUR HEAD, SECURING IT
WITH A BARRETTE, AND
LETTING IT DRY IN THE SUN.

24

FLOWERS

In the south of France, flowers are truly the guests of honor at a marriage. A great Provençal wedding is awash in intensely fragrant white blooms. In my hometown, guests are given bouquets of flowers to carry around, if they wish. The church is usually decorated with lots of flowers as well, and so is the room in which the reception is held. The couple even attaches veils covered with flowers to the cars that ferry guests from the church to the reception.

Have a theme for the flowers. Chose a couple of colors or, even better, a couple of flowers, en masse. Make a statement with the abundance of the flowers, not their variety. And consider the flowers as you choose the colors of other elements within the wedding. For instance, pick candles that complement or blend with the flowers in some way.

If you're getting married in the country, the flowers should be local and in season. Nothing is more pretentious than hothouse flowers in a rustic setting. What could be more attractive than cherry branches, poppies, peonies, roses, lilies of the valley, even sunflowers? Pick one kind, and just go to town with them.

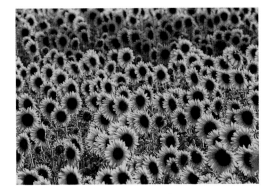

RIGHT: MIXING FOLIAGE WITH THE FLOWERS IN YOUR NUPTUAL
BOUQUET MAKES IT LESS FORMAL, MORE MODERN.

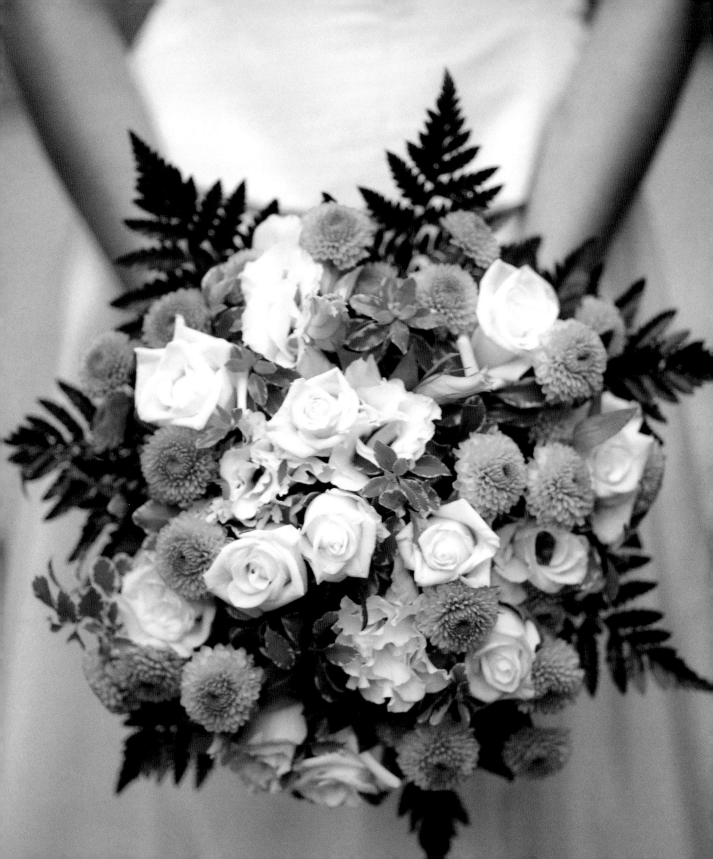

Punctuality is the politeness of kings.
—LOUIS XVIII

25

26

BE IN A GOOD MOOD: IT'S CONTAGIOUS. SMILE AND SAY HELLO TO PIZZA-DELIVERY MEN, DOORMEN, PARKING LOT ATTENDANTS, AND LITTLE OLD LADIES.

USE A SPECIAL JEWELRY CLEANING PRODUCT TO CLEAN YOUR WATCH AS WELL AS YOUR JEWELRY TO MAKE THEM SPARKLE.

27

MEN'S STYLE

For American men, the barber is a beloved mythical figure. The hairstylist, on the other hand, is regarded with suspicion: American men are afraid of being thought of as effeminate if they go to a salon. They want to be perceived as rough and tough. Recently, though, men have begun to realize that a good haircut can facilitate social contact. Men are more vain than women, and a good haircut can really boost a man's fragile ego!

I work with men often at my salons. More and more, they are coming in for treatments as well as for cuts or the occasional highlighting. What is especially gratifying to me is that many of our male clients are receptive to some subtle style pointers; they don't simply bury their heads in a magazine and wait for the ordeal to be over!

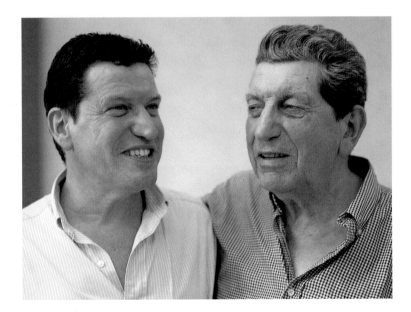

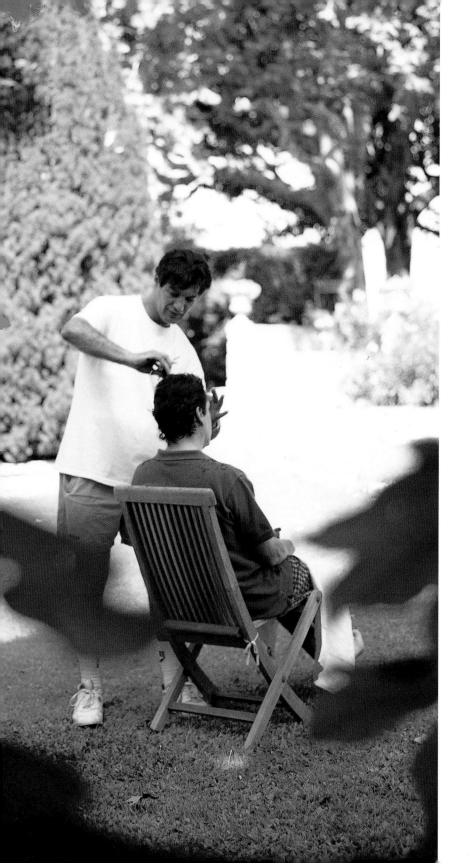

STYLE NOTES

* Don't get locked into a haircut that requires blow-drying.

* If your hairline is receding, wear your hair shorter, a little messier, not too "done."

* Make sure the hair at the nape of your neck tapers gradually; a harsh line is ugly.

* Don't cover your gray hair.

* Trim your sideburns right at cheekbone level, just above the earlobe.

* Keep everything else trimmed as well: ears, brows, nose, mustache, beard.

* Moisturize your skin.

* Don't assume that low-slung pants are sexy.

* Keep your shoes polished.

* Choose clothes in colors that flatter your skin tone.

* Avoid gray, black, or navy shirts for business.

* Find a tailor who will be on your case and won't let you wear something that doesn't fit you.

28 KEEP A SUN HAT IN THE BACKSEAT OF YOUR CAR.

29 **BUY A PAIR OF HOOP EARRINGS**—THEY ARE SO PRETTY WITH A SUMMER DRESS AND A TAN.

30 **REPLACE PHOTOGRAPHS IN FRAMES** TO GIVE YOUR MANTEL A NEW LOOK.

Some men like short hair, others prefer it long. I always encourage my male clients to bring in pictures of cuts they like, as with everyone else. However, a haircut can never cover up a bald spot. Nor for that matter should one try to compensate for hair loss with extra, unnecessary length. It is far better to concentrate on getting a great cut.

The key is proportion. Men need volume in the right places—especially if there is not a great deal of hair to work with. Many stylists cut to create volume at the top, and this is almost always wrong. More volume at the sides balances a man's face and takes the emphasis away from the top of his head, where the perceived problem usually is.

Changing a man's part can help with balance, too. Often men part their hair too low, which can make them look lopsided, even silly: If you point a finger at the iris of one eye, and then bring it up toward your hairline, that's a great spot for a part for practically everyone.

Young men can look great in long hair; it can be very sexy, full of energy. But once you're past forty, shorter is better, especially if you've got even a hint of a receding hairline. It needn't be military short and stiff; even men in conservative professions can get away with hair that's a little messy and tousled as long as it's on the shorter side.

The way a man's hair is cut across the back is crucial. Many stylists cut the hair straight across, which just looks terrible. The edge should be finished in a natural, not-at-all severe way.

Last but not least, hair color for men should never be about covering gray, unless a man has gone dramatically and prematurely white and he doesn't like it. In such a case, we'd put a light gloss of color in, turn it gray-er, a bit less bright. Blond men might use hair color to add some great surfer highlights, but never cover gray.

RIGHT: A CLEAN, CONSERVATIVE HAIRCUT CAN LOOK VERY MODERN AND SEXY WHEN SLIGHTLY TOUSLED.

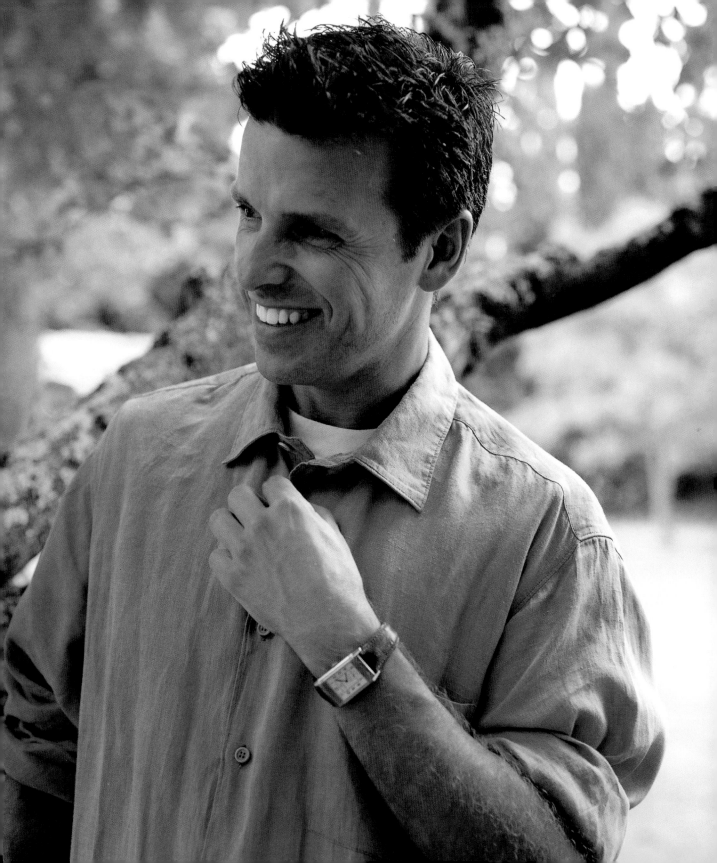

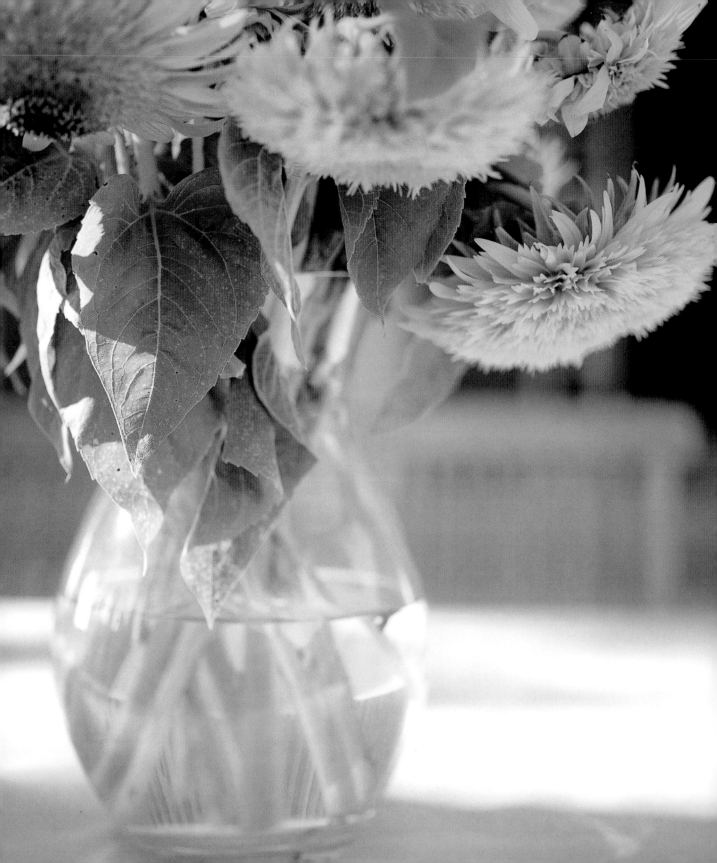

JULY

SUMMER CHIC

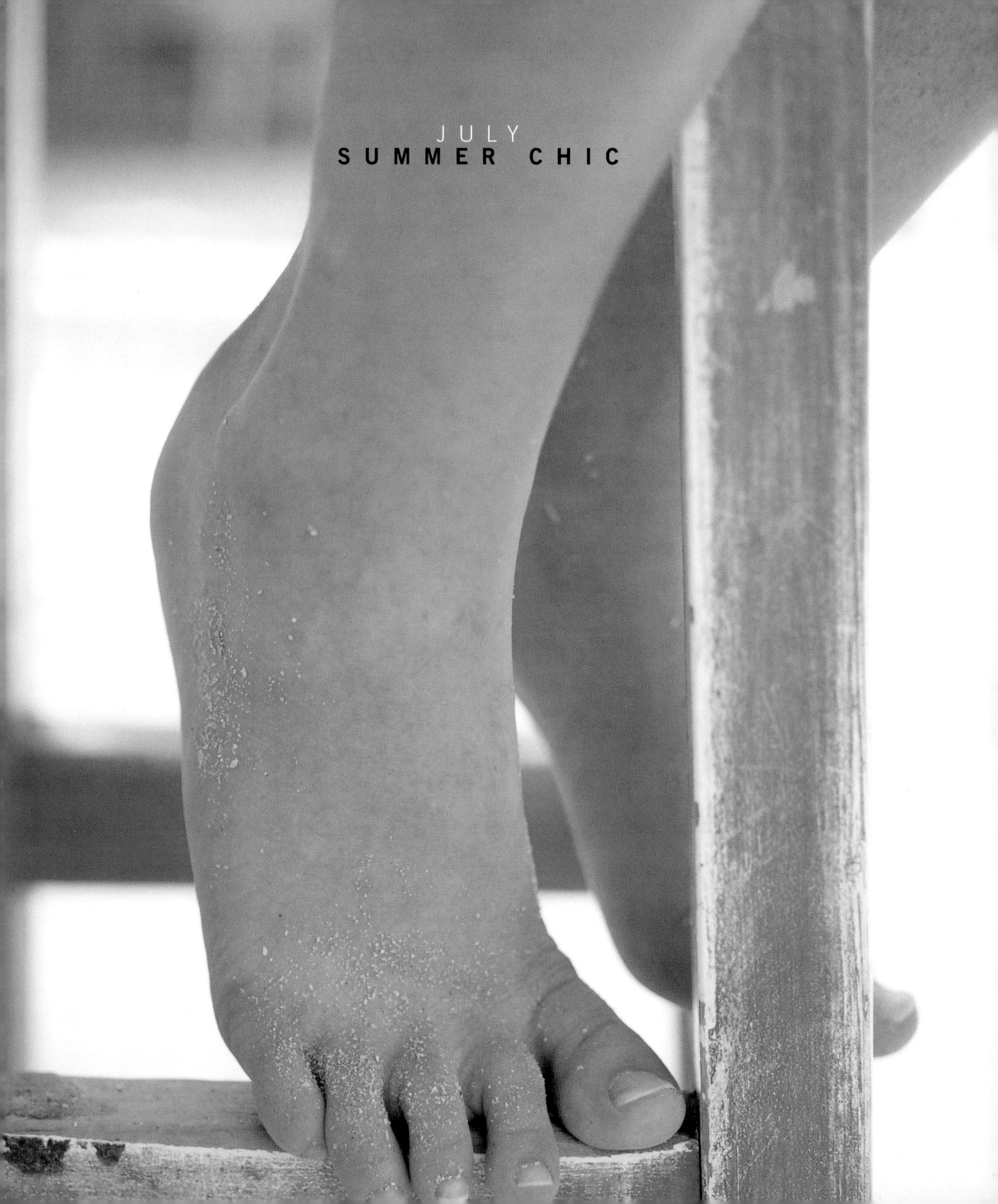

1 **THINK ABOUT GETTING A GREAT WASH-AND-WEAR CUT.** USE FINISHING CREAMS AND POMADES TO CREATE SHINE AND DEFINITION.

2 NOW THAT FRESH VEGETABLES ARE IN SEASON, **TRY TO EAT LOCALLY GROWN ORGANIC PRODUCE.**

3 GIVE YOURSELF PERMISSION TO **TAKE NAPS ONCE IN A WHILE** DURING THE SUMMER. IT IS A TRADITION IN PROVENCE—EVERYONE RESTS AFTER LUNCH WITH THE SHUTTERS CLOSED TO KEEP THE HOUSE COOL.

As soon as the weather gets warm, you want to kick off your shoes and walk barefoot on the beach, at the edge of the surf. How liberating it is to leave a trail of fresh footsteps on wet sand! As waves caress your feet, you rediscover the pleasure of flexing your muscles and the freedom of moving naturally.

July Fourth signals the beginning of a season of great informal parties. With all the doors and windows of your house open, the boundaries between indoors and outdoors are blurred, and your guests can circulate freely without ever feeling like they have to be on their best behavior. It's a perfect occasion to invite intimate friends and their children as well as members of your family. As people mingle or gather in small groups— parents talking about their kids, teens huddling in corners, toddlers running in all directions, young adults checking each other out—you can't help but recall some of your favorite childhood memories.

RIGHT: SUMMER CHIC IS ALL ABOUT THE RIGHT ACCESSORIES AND A RELAXED ATTITUDE.

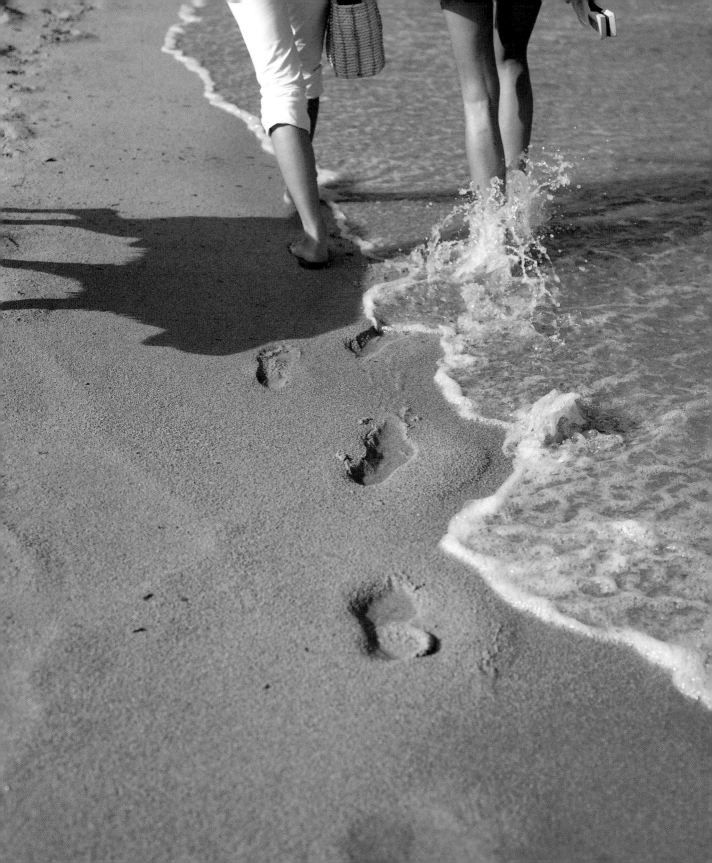

HAPPY FEET

In July pretty feet are a concern for everyone. On Fridays, as people are getting ready to go away for the weekend, it's almost impossible to get a pedicure appointment—every nail expert in the country is booked for the day. But vanity is not the only reason to try to get a pedicure; few things in life are as relaxing as feeling groomed down to your toes.

And while I wouldn't advise getting a pedicure if your weekend plans involve major gardening or house remodeling, I certainly would recommend one before a beach outing, a garden party, a romantic escape, or even a solitary retreat in a mountain cabin. I promise that you'll get great personal satisfaction from stretching your bare legs in front of you, crossing your ankles, and gazing admiringly at your manicured extremities!

* **DON'T EVER LET A PEDICURIST** cut the skin on your feet, or scrape them with razors. It's illegal, it's painful, and it's unnecessary. The only exception might be a hangnail. But cutting cuticles is wrong. If your feet soak long enough, it will be easy to push them back with an orange stick or a towel.

* **A SCRUB,** on the other hand, feels incredible, and gets rid of rough skin and calluses. Scrubs with shea butter in them moisturize and exfoliate the skin at the same time.

* **TO LEAVE YOUR FEET EVEN SOFTER,** rub them at night with a lotion or cream formulated with alphahydroxy acids. Sleep with your socks on.

* **THINK ABOUT THE SHOES YOU'LL BE WEARING.** Wear pale polish with ornate or high-heeled shoes to show off their sexy shape. Plainer shoes with little or no heel can be spiced up with sultry darker polishes. Orange, coral, and fuchsia look rich paired with white or brown shoes.

If you can't get professional help, don't panic. Though you may not think so, your feet are probably fine. As any pedicurist will tell you, everyone believes their feet are awful, so join the club.

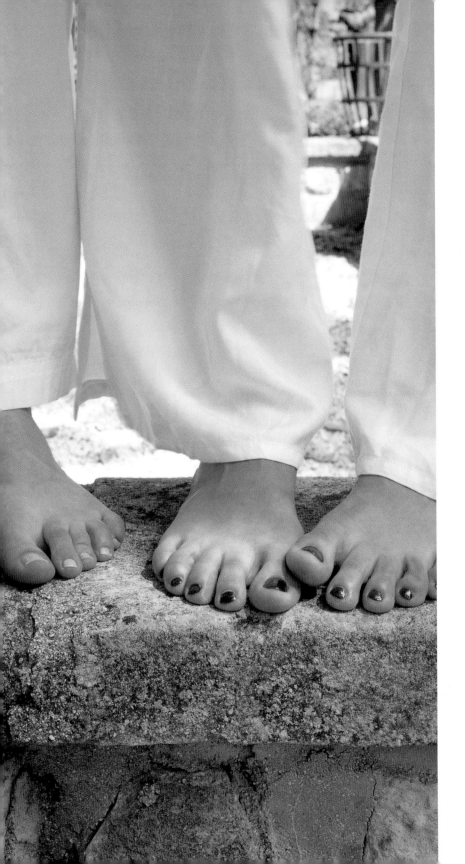

FOOT NOTES

Follow these rules when selecting polish for toes:

∗ DARK REDS, from deep ruby to dark crimson, are drop-dead elegant, while at the same time sexy. Wear them to make a memorable impression.

∗ PALER COLORS, including white, pastels, and seashell shades play up your tan and highlight your carefree attitude.

∗ ORANGE, CORAL, OR FUCHSIA do wonders for very dark skin, but you should avoid them if your complexion is fair.

∗ SORRY, BUT TRENDY COLORS like green, blue, or black are too severe for the most part.

∗ DON'T ALWAYS USE THE SAME polish color on feet and hands.

∗ AND DON'T FORGET that unpolished but well-manicured feet can be beautiful, just by themselves.

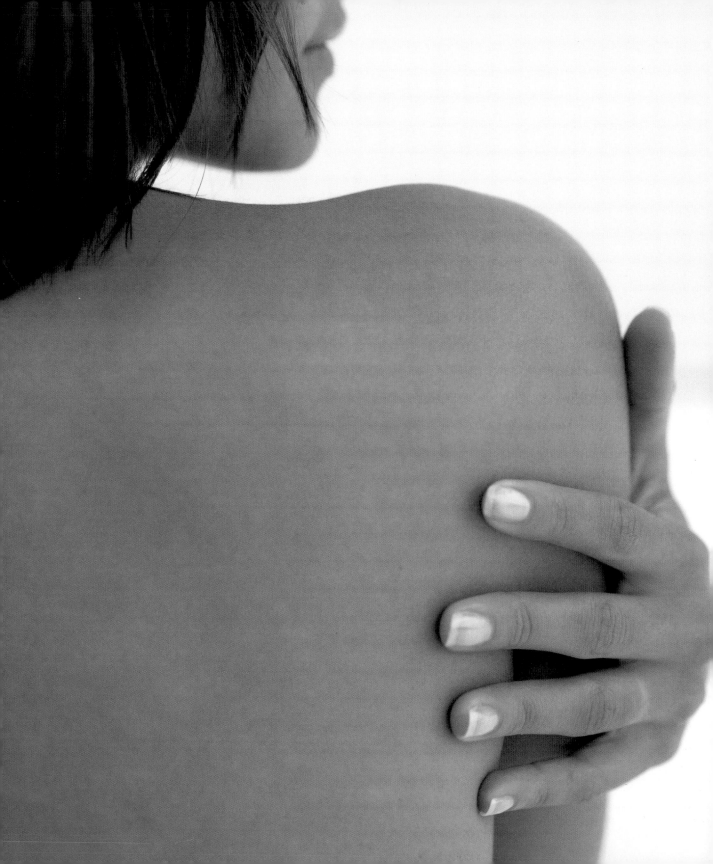

HANDS AND NAILS

While brilliant colors are perfectly appropriate on toes, they often look common on hands. In the evening, choose for your hands a clean red or a subtle shade of burgundy, dusty rose, or burnt orange. If you are wearing a red outfit or gown, don't match your nail polish with it. Keep a safe distance between the two colors.

During the day, pale, sheer polish, or transparent neutrals should be your first choice. I can think of only very few special daytime occasions—maybe a luncheon in an ultra-chic French restaurant or an afternoon film premiere in Hollywood—when wearing pink, coral, or red nail polish on your hands is attractive. So be ruthless in the morning; remove the colorful polish you wore the night before at that fancy charity ball or wild birthday party. Let's face it, a woman who displays a garish daytime manicure—even if she is tastefully dressed and beautifully groomed—looks a bit tacky.

* **ARTIFICIAL NAILS,** silk wraps, tips—just don't go there. They weaken your nails, and they can cause all kinds of nail problems and even diseases.
* **KEEP YOUR NAILS ROUND OR SQUARE.** A subtle version of either is fine; anything severe looks strange.
* **PUSH BACK CUTICLES** with a towel after you shower instead of cutting them, which dries them out, irritates them, and creates hangnails.
* **KEEP A LITTLE OIL** (scented or not) by your bed or desk to keep cuticles soft.
* **IF YOUR LIFESTYLE ALLOWS YOU TO HAVE LONG NAILS,** and you can achieve them without artificial nails, fine. But if you love gardening, have small children, go rock-climbing . . . short is as chic, if not more so.
* **FOR SUMMER NAILS,** I think women look great with just a touch of barely-there, pale cream polish, almost as if the nails have only been buffed.
* **CHIPPED POLISH LOOKS AWFUL.** To keep polish from chipping, apply it in thin coats and go over the polish every few days with a clear topcoat.
* **A BASE COAT** will keep polish from staining your nails.

TREAT A FRIEND TO LUNCH FOLLOWED BY A MANICURE AT YOUR FAVORITE SALON FOR HER BIRTHDAY.

7

CHILL GLASSES FOR SUMMER BEVERAGES.

8

USE A MOISTURIZING SHEA BUTTER SOAP TO PREVENT DRY SUMMER SKIN.

9

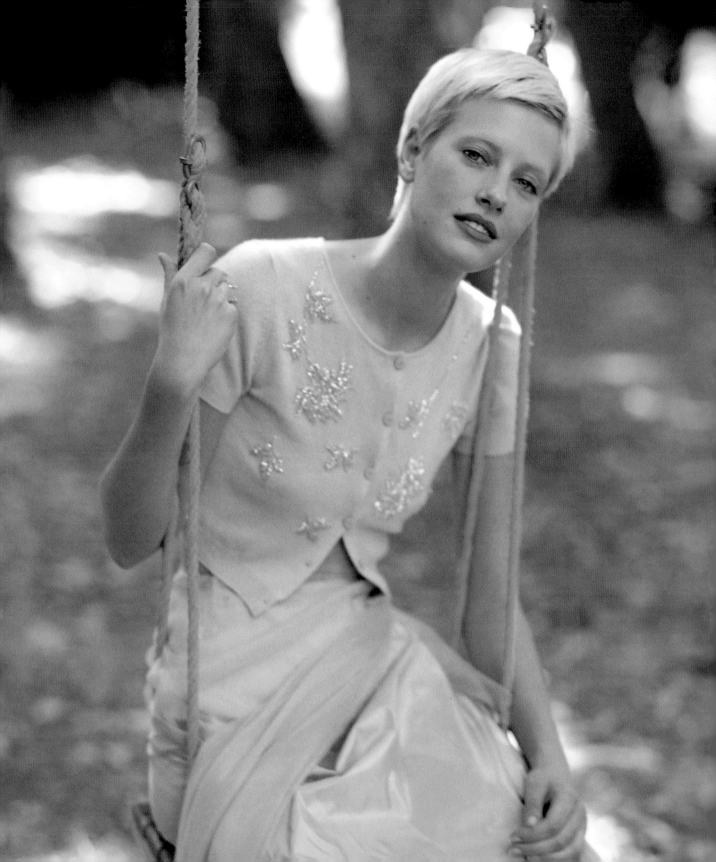

FREE AND EASY SUMMER HAIR

If the catchword for July is "freedom," let it extend to your hair as well. Now is the time for the very simplest of styles. Who can fuss with a blow-dry, styling, and products when the ocean beckons and the mercury is climbing. The biggest complaint I hear in the summer is frizzy hair. The thing is, when it's really humid and hot outside, it's important that the hair be natural—a big blow-dry every day is just not right.

* **OVERLY COIFFED HAIR** looks out of place in the middle of summer. Find a style that looks free and easy.
* **YOUR HAIR DOES GROW FASTER IN THE SUMMER,** so get it trimmed a little more often and you'll be in great shape. To avoid frizz, though, make sure your cut doesn't have lots of layers.
* **IF YOUR HAIR FRIZZES** anyway, use gel, styling cream, and hair accessories to keep it under control.
* **IF YOU HAVE A REAL MOP OF WILD CURLS,** put tons of cream on it when it's wet, and let it dry in a ponytail.

To control the summer frizzies, many of my clients try to fight the natural texture of their hair. It's a mistake, a sure way to wage a losing battle against humidity. It's much more modern, and a lot more practical, to accept the texture of your hair, even to play it up. In the long run, doing so is always more flattering and less time-consuming.

Before deciding on the form of a cut, regardless of the season, I first evaluate the texture of a client's hair. It's a matter of common sense. In architecture, the texture of a stone will determine the way it is carved. In carpentry, the texture of a piece of wood will define how it is trimmed. In fashion, the texture of a fabric will dictate the way it is cut.

LEFT: THIS SHORT, CAREFREE CUT IS GREAT FOR SUMMER. IT'S COOL AND CHIC AND REQUIRES VERY LITTLE MAINTENANCE.

PREPARE YOUR WEEKEND **BAG** ON THURSDAY FOR A QUICK FRIDAY GETAWAY. TUCK IN SOME SACHETS.

10

BUY A BIG SQUARE PIECE **OF PROVENÇAL FABRIC** TO HEM FOR AN IMPROMPTU PICNIC CLOTH.

11

EVEN WHEN YOU HAVE A LIGHT TAN, **CREAM BLUSH ON THE APPLE OF YOUR CHEEKS** WILL MAKE YOU LOOK PRETTIER.

12

MAKE MOROCCAN ICED TEA BY MIXING MINT TEA WITH ORANGE JUICE. SERVE OVER ICE. USE ORANGE SLICES AS A GARNISH.

13

BASTILLE DAY: **HANG PAPER LANTERNS IN YOUR PATIO** AND INVITE NEIGHBORS TO A "LET-THEM-EAT-CAKE" AFTER-DINNER DANCE PARTY.

14

SLICK YOUR HAIR BACK WITH HAIR CREAM WHEN IT'S STILL DAMP INSTEAD OF BLOW-DRYING IT. YOU'LL SAVE TIME AND STILL LOOK POLISHED.

15

CURLY HAIR My rule of thumb is never to choose an everyday hairstyle that doesn't work with your natural hair texture. Unfortunately, most women with a curly mane wish they had straight hair. Little do they know that most women with straight hair wish they had some curls. *C'est la vie!*

While I would agree that blowing your hair straight can create a glamorous evening look that works for almost everyone—particularly if you want to show off at a formal event—it is extremely labor-intensive. If you had to do it every morning, you would have to get up an hour earlier. Sleep is much too important to health and beauty to squander it on such a trivial pursuit.

There are so many gorgeous hairstyles for curly hair, it is a shame not to take advantage of them. Work with your hairstylist to come up with a few different styles, so you aren't always locked into one look.

THE GOOD NEWS:

* **YOU'VE GOT GREAT NATURAL TEXTURE AND SUPPORT.** Putting your hair up is easier; styles will stay in place better.
* **CURLY HAIR,** once the frizz is controlled, can look just gorgeous when long.
* **A CHIN-LENGTH BOB** is very elegant for curly or wavy hair, but you'll definitely need finishing cream to smooth out the curls, and often some clips at the sides. Comb some texturizing balm through the hair when it's still wet, then part the hair to the side. Think '20s or '30s, and dress with that in mind.
* **A GREAT WAY TO GET SOME HEIGHT** at the roots is to tie a bandanna from the back of the neck to the top of the hairline; it's a modern version of a '30s hairstyle. Or try a wide headband and think of Audrey Hepburn! You can run out with it still wet, and it always looks fresh.

THE BAD NEWS:

* **YOUR MAIN ENEMY,** particularly during the summer, is frizz. It is best controlled with texturizing balms and straightening or finishing creams.

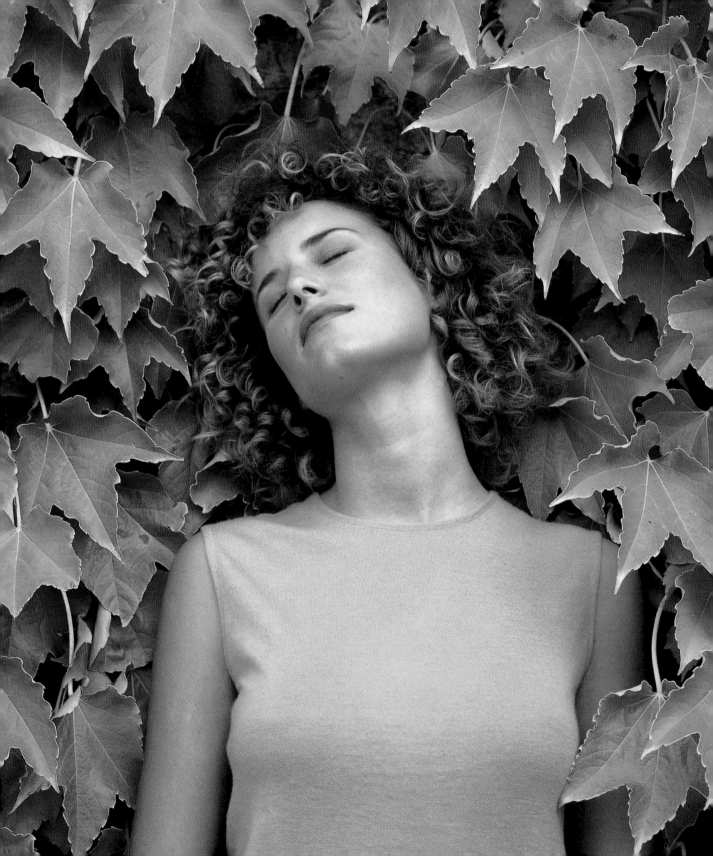

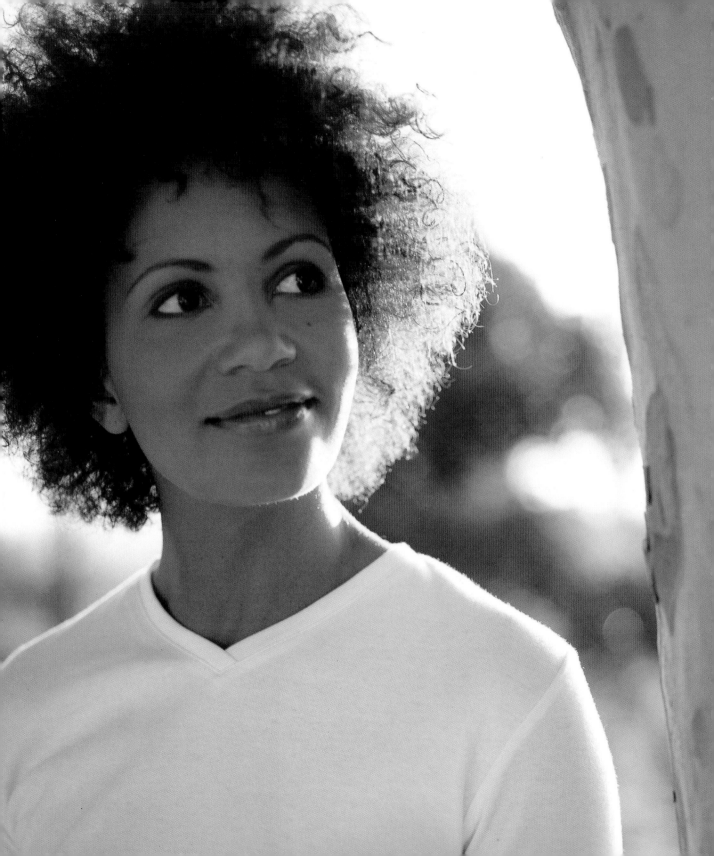

* **BRUSHING YOUR HAIR** distributes air through it, creating more frizz. So always use a bit of finishing cream or balm on the ends after you brush dry hair.
* **BEWARE OF LAYERS,** whether you plan to leave your hair curly or blow it straight. Layers tempt the hair to curl upward more quickly, creating volume where you don't want it, not to mention the dreaded frizz.

AFRICAN-AMERICAN HAIR Black women's hair texture requires a different sort of effort than Caucasian or Asian hair. It can be so incredible-looking whether it's straightened or left curly; the thing to avoid with most black hair is layers. And don't fight the texture (unless you can afford to have a stylist work on you virtually every day).

Jane, one of my favorite clients, is somewhere in her fifties, but if you told me she was just turning thirty, I'd believe you. "That's one of the great things about black skin," she says, when people exclaim over how young she looks. "It ages much better." Over the years, we've settled on a great, chin-length bob for Jane, a length that allows her to wear it naturally, in a modified Afro shape, or straightened, glossy, and smooth. We cut Jane's hair shorter in the summer, so she can wear it curly more often.

* **BLACK HAIR IS DEFINITELY MORE DELICATE;** it breaks easily, so loads of conditioner (I especially recommend shea butter) is very important.
* **TO GET IT STRAIGHT,** smooth, and flat, blow-dry your hair using either a flat or rounded brush, depending on the look you are after.
* **ON STRAIGHTENED HAIR,** texturizing and finishing creams are a must, but too much will look greasy.
* **BLACK WOMEN WITH LONG HAIR,** whether natural or straightened, often look fantastic in a ponytail.
* **BLACK HAIR IS IDEAL FOR HAIR ACCESSORIES:** they stay in better than they do in Caucasian or Asian hair, and they show up well against the dark brown or black of the hair.

USE CITRONELLA CANDLES AS AN INSECT REPELLENT. ADDED BONUS: THEIR SCENT IS SOOTHING IF YOU ARE PRONE TO HEADACHES OR MIGRAINES.

16

KEEP SUMMER SHOES POLISHED. DUSTY SANDALS AND LOAFERS LOOK TERRIBLE.

17

GOT A NEW HAIRCUT AND HATE IT? DON'T FRET. CHANGE THE COLOR OF YOUR LIPSTICK INSTEAD. A BRIGHTER SHADE WILL BRING OUT THE CHARACTER OF YOUR FACE AND MAKE THE CUT LESS IMPORTANT.

18

BUY VINTAGE POSTCARDS AND SEND THEM TO FRIENDS YOU NORMALLY ONLY E-MAIL OR PHONE.

19

IMPROVISE A SUMMER FILM FESTIVAL BY INVITING YOUR FRIENDS TO WATCH FOREIGN FILMS, DOCUMENTARIES, OR ART FILMS.

20

MAKE TURKISH-STYLE GRILLED CHICKEN MARINATED IN YOGURT AND FRESH CUMIN SEEDS.

21

STRAIGHT HAIR Women with super-straight hair, who for so long worried endlessly about volume, are in luck: Straight and flat requires very little work, and looks elegant with a little grooming.

If you've got an oval face, though, you'll definitely want some layers, at least around the face, to get that perfect amount of volume at the sides. A blunt cut, on the other hand, will give you fullness at the bottom.

* **A SHORT CUT** will almost always need layers: Straight and short can look like a little hat instead of a haircut. Highlights can also help break things up a bit.
* **THINK ABOUT PUTTING YOUR HAIR UP** if it's going to be exceptionally hot and sticky, as straight hair can get stringy in these conditions. Straight hair makes beautiful, neat ponytails, and great braids.
* **YOU CAN USE A SMALL BARRETTE** to create a bit of volume and interest at the sides, just the way layers might: The line of the pulled-back hair also creates a sort of visual break-point.
* **CURLING IRONS CAN FRY YOUR HAIR,** and the little tiny curls they create often look out of place against the rest of your hair. If you must have curl, rollers—or even just a blow-dry with a round brush—are a better route, as they create a sense of curl throughout the hair, rather than in one, odd little spot.
* **DON'T LET ANYONE TALK YOU INTO GETTING A PERM.** There's nothing more unnatural-looking. Not only will it leave your hair smelling foul, it will also make it dry and porous.

KEEPING HAIR LOOKING GREAT, ALL SUMMER

During the summer, no matter what type of hair you have, chlorine, sun, and salt can be murder on it: If you are not careful, dull-looking hair, split ends, and yellow or brassy-looking highlights are to be expected.

Chlorine, in particular, can wreak havoc with hair color, especially highlights and other kinds of color involving bleach. Hair that turns green from

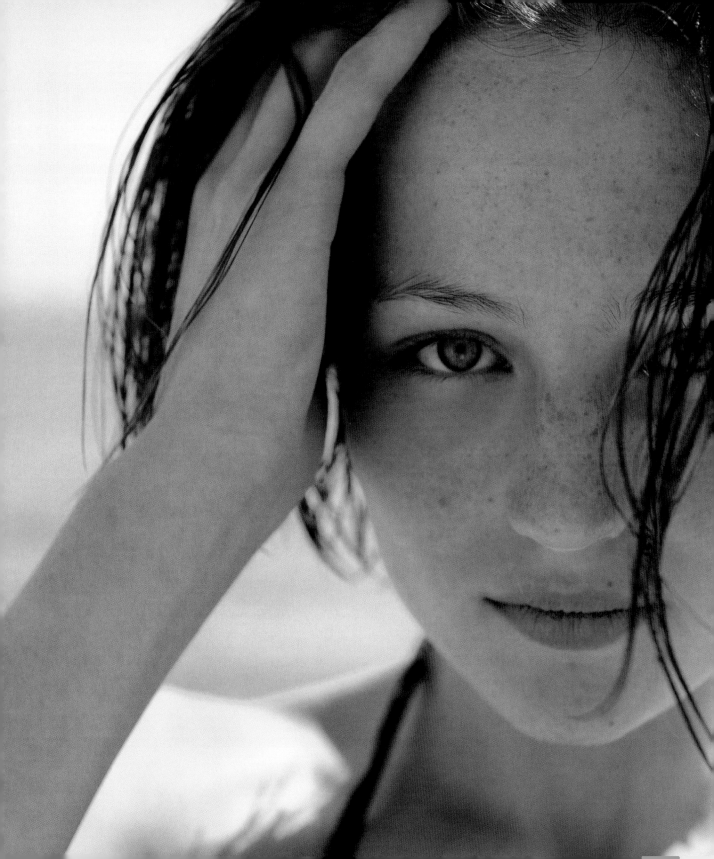

MOISTURIZING HAIR

Summer is a time to moisturize your hair with masks, shea butter in particular. Before jumping in the swimming pool, protect your hair from chlorine by rubbing a moisturizing agent in it. Or try an application of olive oil to revive hair damaged by sun and surf. Apply on dry hair. Wear it all day under a scarf or a hat. As everyone in Provence will tell you, olive oil is a miracle beauty product for both hair and skin.

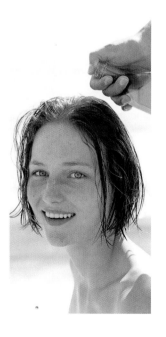

chlorine has generally suffered from too many chemical processes, so it's become porous. Once it is green, there isn't a great deal to be done except to put in a semi-permanent color rinse, which will mask the greenish tint.

While it's possible to fix these problems, the best strategy is to avoid summer-stressed hair altogether. Protect your hair to the maximum.

* Before you go in the pool, slick on conditioner or a hair mask or use a bathing cap, though that's rarely the most ideal look for anyone.
* Once you're out, rinse, rinse, rinse, using a rinsing agent, like apple cider mixed with water, to help things along. Then condition again.
* In the sun, or when swimming in salt water, do much the same thing: Use lots of conditioner (one with sunscreen if possible), combined with a hat.

SUMMER SKIN CARE

The heat, humidity, and, in some cases, extreme dryness of summertime air has aestheticians working overtime as soon as July comes around. You do need to change your skin care with the seasons, or at least make slight adjustments. A facial once a month during the summer can take care of most weather-related problems.

OILY SKIN Oily skin is at its worst at this time of year: Increased heat and humidity cause oil production to increase. Sweat, chemicals in sunscreens, and plain old heat can cause acne flare-ups, even in skin that normally doesn't break out. To control oily skin, many women use drying preparations, such as toner with alcohol, or harsh, drying acne medications designed for teenage skin. Unfortunately, it is the wrong strategy. The drying agents trick the skin into thinking it's too dry, and encouraging it to produce even more oil.

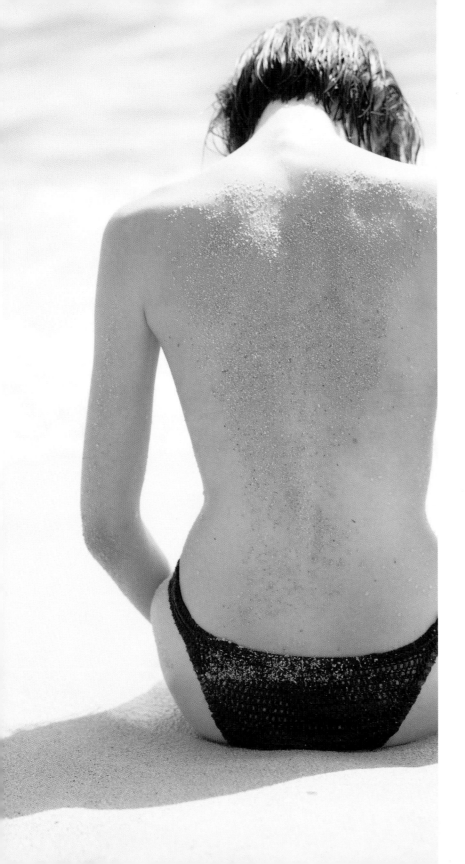

KEEP A PAIR OF SCISSORS IN YOUR GLOVE COMPARTMENT TO CUT WILDFLOWERS ALONG THE ROADSIDE. (BUT BE SURE TO LEAVE SOME FOR OTHERS!)

GROW BASIL IN A POT ALL SUMMER LONG BY KEEPING IT ON A SUNNY WINDOWSILL AND WATERING IT OFTEN.

WHEN THE TEMPERATURE RISES, **SIMPLIFY, SIMPLIFY.** YOU DON'T HAVE TO GET "DRESSED UP" TO HAVE STYLE.

CONSULT WITH YOUR FACIALIST TO SEE IF YOU NEED TO MODIFY YOUR MOISTURIZING ROUTINE.

25

WORK OUT BAREFOOT OCCASIONALLY TO STRENGTHEN THE SMALL MUSCLES IN YOUR FEET.

26

WAXING IS LESS PAINFUL WHEN DONE REGULARLY, SO SCHEDULE MONTHLY APPOINT-MENTS ALL YEAR LONG, NOT JUST IN THE WARMER MONTHS.

27

The best strategy is not to panic, and not to overcleanse your skin. Instead, treat your skin with a product that contains one of the following ingredients:

* **SALICYLIC ACID** that treats both existing breakouts and prevents new ones.
* **TEA TREE OIL,** a natural anti-inflammatory and antibacterial agent that smells rather bad but clears up problems quickly.
* **VITAMIN C SERUMS** that heal breakouts and prevent new ones at the same time.
* **OLIVE OIL SOAP** that's gentle yet not oily. The main ingredient of a French soap called Savon de Marseilles, olive oil replenishes skin's natural moisture while the soap cleanses it. Olive oil soap works miracles against blemishes.
* **TO REMOVE EXTRA OIL FROM YOUR SKIN,** blot the problem area with a tissue or with blotter papers, then lightly dust on some translucent powder.

If your skin really causes trouble, don't hesitate to consult a dermatologist: Between topical and oral antibiotics, most breakout problems can be dealt with successfully. If this is an emergency—let's say you have to be on television the next day—many dermatologists will give you a shot of cortisone that will get rid of a blemish overnight.

DRY SKIN In hot and humid climates, your dry skin is likely to get a break, but in dry places, like Arizona, New Mexico, or L.A., its dryness can increase. To control flakiness due to dryness, try the following:

* **USE A MOISTURIZING SUNSCREEN,** and apply it often; once in the morning and once in the afternoon, and as many times as you want in between.
* **CLEANSE** with the gentlest of cleansers, only at night.
* **APPLY** only moisturizing foundations and lipsticks.
* **DRINK** glasses upon glasses of water.
* **BUY** a humidifier.

EXFOLIATION Your skin used to exfoliate itself perfectly well when you were a child. As we age, the exfoliation process slows down. As a result, dead skin cells linger on top of the skin, making it look dull, patchy, or flaky. Exfoliating your skin regularly will make it brighter, more vital-looking, even younger. If you use self-tanners, regular use of exfoliators will make your artificial tan much smoother and natural-looking. There are two choices when it comes to exfoliating skin: physical or chemical exfoliators.

* **A PHYSICAL EXFOLIATOR** is basically a good scrub. You can exfoliate with anything from a rough washcloth or a loofah, to sea salt, apricot kernel grains, herbs . . . anything rough enough to get rid of dead cells. If your skin is oily or sensitive, though, don't scrub it. The mechanical action of exfoliators can irritate the epidermis and cause flare-ups.
* **CHEMICAL EXFOLIATORS** include alphahydroxy acids, some vitamin C serums, and some vitamin A–based products, from over-the-counter retinol creams to prescription-only creams like Retin-A and Renova. Always use these in conjunction with a regular regimen of sunscreens.

SHAVING OR WAXING? At the beginning of the bathing-suit season, everyone thinks about removing unwanted hair—hardly a pleasurable prospect, no matter what method you choose.

* **BECAUSE HAIR GROWTH** is stimulated by shaving, unless you shave every day, your legs will never look smooth and satiny.
* **WAXING** would be the perfect solution if it wasn't so painful. Green wax, pink wax, honey wax, sugar wax—they all hurt to some extent or another. But legs are such beautiful parts of the body, why not go the distance and make them even more seductive. Experiment and find an aesthetician you like, then book a regular schedule, especially in the summer months.
* **LASER TREATMENTS** that promise to remove hair permanently are costly and aren't yet that effective: At the most, the effects last about a year.

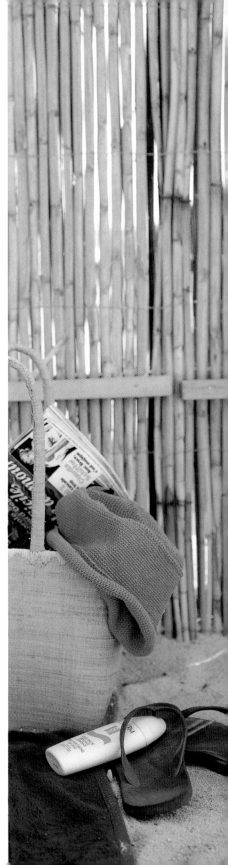

CITRON PRESSÉ

Citron pressé means in French "pressed lemon." A lemon is squeezed—or pressed—directly into your glass and sugar and water are added.

But because this typical French lemonade doesn't contain as much sugar as its American counterpart, you drink it very slowly, one dainty sip at a time. The *citron pressé* is an anti-stress concoction. Needless to say, it's a popular drink in Provence, where people are proud of their leisurely, laid-back lifestyle.

When in Aix, don't order a pressed lemon if you are pressed for time!

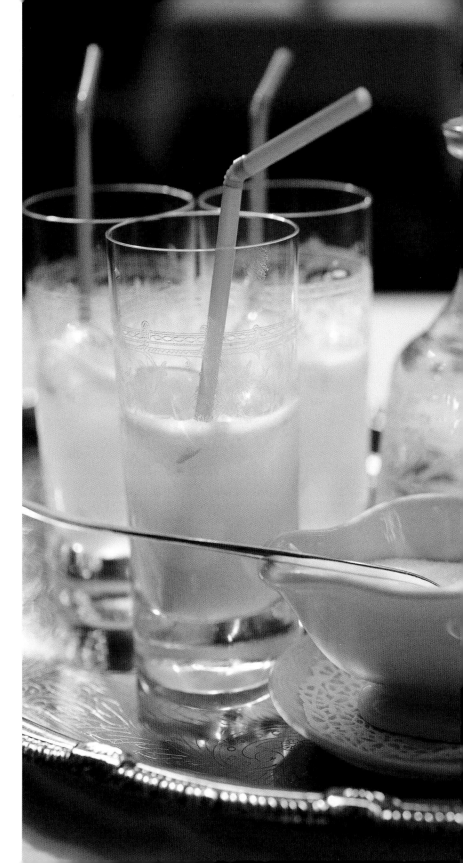

SUN AND SKIN CARE There are few things sexier than a strappy summer dress sliding off a bronzed shoulder, but take care before you head out into the bright light of day. In July the sun's rays really are more powerful than just a month ago, and while temperatures may not be at their summer highs, it might as well be August as far as your skin is concerned.

Though you should always be prepared to deal with the sun, you should also try to avoid being exposed to it for more than a few minutes. Think of a sunscreen as something you wear just in case—if you have no choice but to sit in the sun; if you must go shopping in an open market; if you want to sit through a tennis match; if you must cross a scorching parking lot to get to your car. Choose an SPF 15 or higher for effective protection.

The presence of the sun in the environment is exhilarating, but you get more benefits from it if you stay at a safe distance, in the cool shade of a tree, under an umbrella, or under the awning at the terrace of a café. The narrow streets of my native town were designed to be shady, with the buildings placed in such a way as to protect passersby from the harsh rays of the Provençal sun.

Beyond sunscreens and sunblocks, think about hats, umbrellas, and, my favorite, beach outings at dawn or sunset. Enjoy the heat but not the rays of the sun—don't jeopardize your future health.

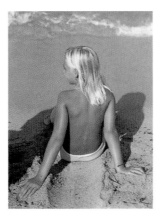

BUY CLOTHES MADE OF 80 PERCENT LINEN AND 20 PERCENT COTTON: THEY WILL BE BOTH COOL AND WRINKLE-RESISTANT.

28

IF YOU CAN'T GO AWAY FOR A SUMMER VACATION, AT LEAST **BOOK A WEEKEND PACKAGE AT A LUXURY RESORT AND SPA** IN YOUR AREA.

29

RENT A SPORTY RED CONVERTIBLE FOR A WEEKEND GETAWAY, EVEN IF YOU ALREADY HAVE A CAR.

30

BUY ORGANIC HONEY AND USE IT INSTEAD OF SUGAR.

31

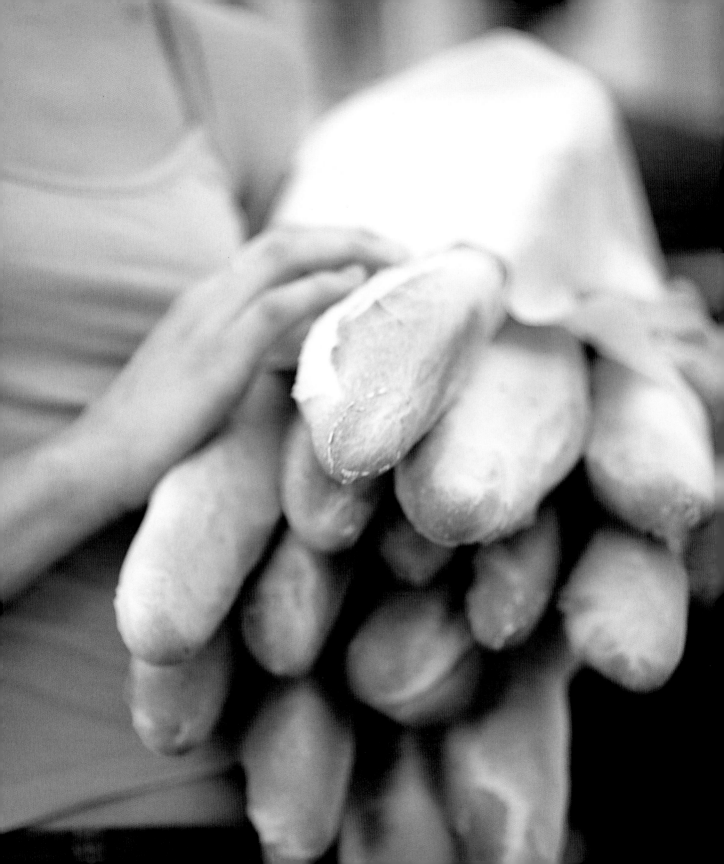

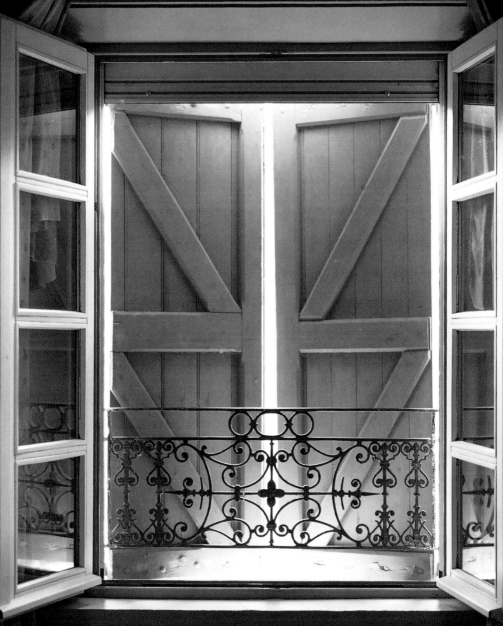

THINK LAVENDER. PICK
FISTFULS FROM YOUR
GARDEN, OR BUY BUNCHES
FROM YOUR FLORIST TO
ARRANGE IN CERAMIC VASES,
TERRA-COTTA FLOWERPOTS,
OLD JAM JARS—ANYTHING.

1

TO DRESS UP A CASUAL
SUMMER OUTFIT, **TIE A
COLORFUL COTTON SCARF**
AROUND YOUR NECK.

2

HAVE A SEA-SALT PEDICURE
TO EXFOLIATE DRY SKIN,
FOLLOWED BY A MOISTUR-
IZING FOOT MASSAGE.

3

Whether or not you take time off from work in August, it is the slowest and the most relaxed period of the year. Of course, Americans are nowhere as laid-back as Europeans, who traditionally go away on vacation from the end of July to September first! Still, even here, business schedules are less frantic and three-day weekends are not uncommon during this last summer month.

It is a time to enjoy life in a leisurely way. For me, this means recon-necting with my roots, my childhood, my role as a father, and sharing with my son the pleasure of an old-fashioned French vacation. Every August, I spend at least three weeks somewhere near Aix-en-Provence, my hometown. There is something particularly relaxing about a vacation in a place you know and love: You don't feel compelled to go out and explore like a tourist. Instead, the discoveries are more incidental, and acciden-tal, like finding an old man making tiles at the end of a little country road, or

RIGHT: I LOVE INTRODUCING MY SON, ALEXANDRE,
TO THE COUNTRYSIDE OF MY CHILDHOOD EACH SUMMER.

page 172

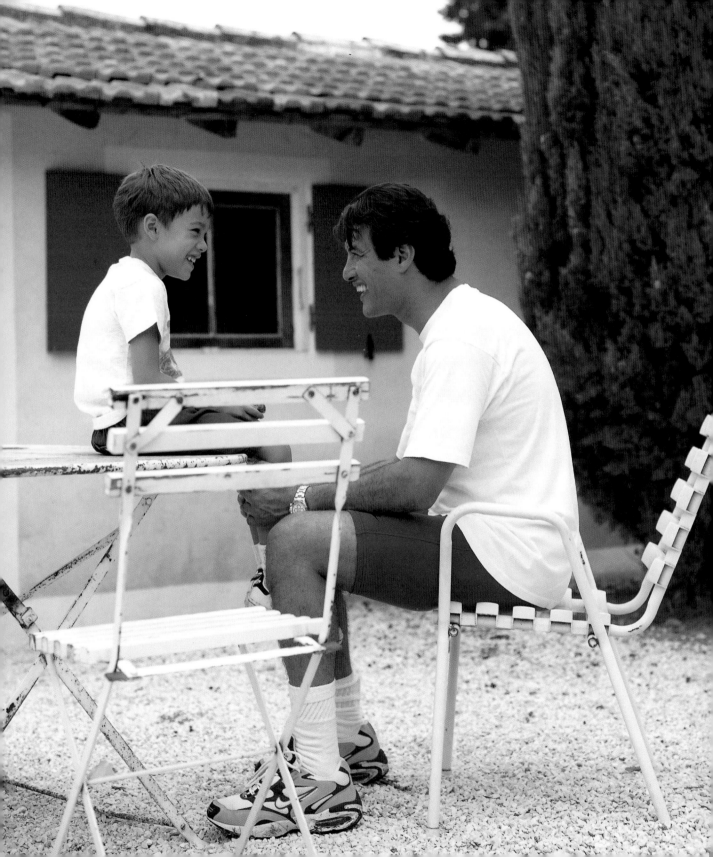

LISTEN TO COOL JAZZ. MILES DAVIS IS THE PERFECT SOUND FOR SULTRY SUMMER NIGHTS.

4

BUY A FUN NEW HAIR ACCESSORY. AUGUST IS DEFINITELY A TIME YOU'LL WANT TO WEAR YOUR HAIR UP.

5

STOP AT A ROADSIDE FARMER'S MARKET AND BUY EXTRA PRODUCE TO SHARE WITH NEIGHBORS OR CO-WORKERS.

6

gathering sunflowers in a friend's field, or shopping at the local outdoor market for whatever happens to strike your fancy.

As a child, I remember wandering through La Place de la Madeleine, a huge square in Aix surrounded by centuries-old plane trees where, to this day, a thriving farmer's market is still held three times a week. The sheer abundance of colors, vegetables, spices, fabrics, crafts, antiques, scents, and textures is just as overwhelming now as it was then. Nothing much has changed: Merchants and their customers banter with each other as they bargain over the price of a kilo of peaches or an ounce of turmeric. Shoppers of both sexes carry colorful straw panniers for their groceries. And the women look incredibly chic in sleeveless cotton dresses, or Capri pants with ballerina flats, their hair neatly caught up with a barrette or anchored casually with a pencil. Their look says: "This is who I am. Don't expect me to be a slave to fashion."

In fact, the materials and colors of my accessory collection were inspired by these memories.

SUMMER STYLE

The South of France, from Provence to the Côte d'Azur, is known the world over for its elegance. Home of the troubadours in the Middle Ages, it is still today a land of grace and poetry. In fact, medieval minstrels from this region are credited with glorifying romantic love in epic poems retelling how chivalrous knights wooed virtuous and noble ladies. Back then, Provence was much more civilized than the northern part of France, and Aix was considered a more sophisticated capital than Paris.

The rivalry between the two cities is legendary. Though Paris is the capital of fashion in winter, during the summer, and particularly in August, Aix is

RIGHT: COLORFUL STRAW BAGS LINED WITH PROVENÇAL FABRIC ARE *THE* INDISPENSABLE SUMMER ACCESSORY.

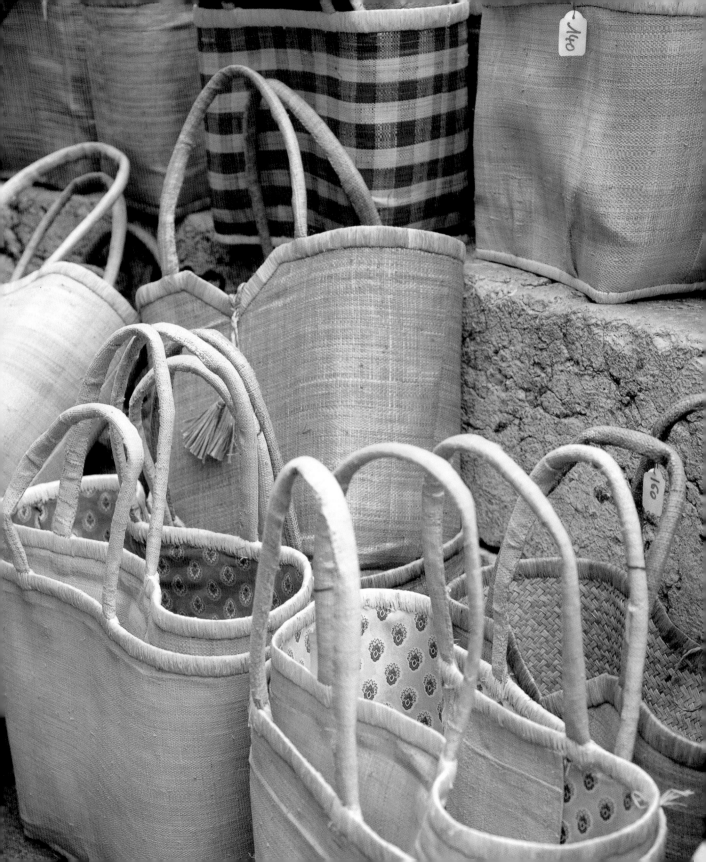

DON'T FORGET TO SCHEDULE
A MONTHLY APPOINTMENT
FOR EYEBROW SHAPING.

the place to see and be seen. The women look like they have strolled out of a 1930 Lartigue photograph: Their attire is timeless yet surprisingly modern, adapted to the weather, the season, and the activity of the moment.

The women of Provence have always inspired me with their incredible sense of style. It's a look of supreme simplicity that my most stylish clients have embraced as well. I don't know if it's the light or the lifestyle, but on the streets of Aix you'll rarely see a woman wearing too much makeup, flashy clothes, an armful of gold jewelry, or tons of hairspray. It just doesn't happen. Here are some typical summer ensembles:

* **A PALE COTTON SHIRTDRESS** with leather mules, or even flip-flops. A great manicure and pedicure. A neat ponytail.
* **BALLET FLATS** with Capri pants, a straw basket in hand. A chic bob, tucked behind the ears, with long bangs.
* **A SIMPLE STRAPPY TOP,** a slim wrap skirt, hair held in place with a single braid. Ah, braided hair! How cool and romantic.
* **A STRIPED TOP** with natural linen slacks. Sunglasses casually propped on the head, like a headband, with a few strands of hair falling down.
* **LIGHT CANVAS PANTS,** a blue plaid or crisp white cotton shirt, a rope belt, espadrilles, and a straw Panama.
* **A COTTON DRESS** with a pashmina scarf, worn with pretty espadrilles. It looks even better if you carry a loaf of bread and a bouquet of flowers!

8 BUY A GREAT FALL HANDBAG
NOW—YOU'LL HAVE MORE
CHOICES.

But these fashion tips won't work unless you add a final personal touch: a taste for the unexpected combined with a sense of whimsy. Needless to say, this isn't something that can be dictated. The only way to learn it is by observing how others do it. This is why in Aix people spend so much time sitting at the terraces of cafés, sipping lemonade, watching the continuous parade of chic local residents, dapper out-of-towners, colorful international tourists, and in-the-know students.

9 CLEAN YOUR SKIN WITH A
SOFT TONER EVERY MORNING
TO KEEP IT BLEMISH-FREE ALL
SUMMER LONG.

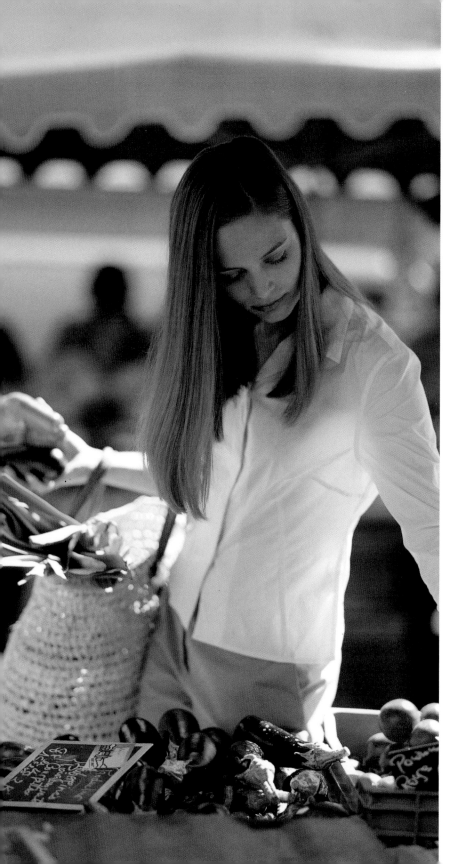

SUMMER ELEGANCE

Here are the principles Provençal women use to put together a summer look that's effortless:

✳ THINK FIRST ABOUT FIT, even with casual clothes: They should be neither too tight nor too loose, but just skimming the body lightly.

✳ AVOID LABELS. Large designer emblems are considered very unchic in the country.

✳ CHOOSE COLORS THAT ARE FOOLPROOF, like navy blue and white. Olive and cream, pink and pale gray, or pale pink and powder blue are other never-miss combinations.

✳ FAVOR SIMPLE, NATURAL FABRICS like cotton and linen. Artificial fibers, which look good in the store, appear coarse and unnatural in the light of day.

✳ EMBRACE KHAKIS. The French know that khakis have enduring style, but they choose those made of very fine fabric. Heavier khakis look like work clothes, and aren't as comfortable.

SUMMER ELEGANCE

(continued)

* **WEAR DRESSES WITH THE LEAST FUSSY SHAPES:** The fabric can be wild as long as the cut is simple and easy.

* **REMEMBER THAT THE TIME** to wear something revealing is at the swimming pool or the beach—and that's it.

* **DEAL GRACEFULLY with** a bad hair day by tying a bandanna or scarf around your head.

* **CONSIGN YOUR BLACK LEATHER BAG** to the closet during the heat of summer. A bag made of straw, colored fabric, or canvas is the French woman's bag of choice from June to September.

* **KEEP YOUR MAKEUP AS SOFT** and barely-there as possible. See page 180 for specifics.

When I go back home, I am always surprised how observant the locals really are. They look relaxed, yet they notice everything. If you get lost and ask for directions, for instance, they will describe in detail the fountains, the clocks, and the trees that will serve as landmarks for you to find your way around. As they talk to you, moving their hands this way and that to indicate which way to turn, they share with you the pleasure of looking at that little bridge, that garden, that statue, that portal, or that old street.

Looking at landscapes, things, or people is the best way to relax and learn at the same time. One of the benefits of this laid-back activity is a greater appreciation of the poetry of life—the key to real style. Indeed, stylists, designers, and decorators are nothing but professional poets, hired to bring serendipity and magic into their client's life. I know so many Wall Street tycoons who spend a lot of money building fantastic mansions. Within this environment, they seek a touch of romance, effortlessness, simplicity—they seek poetry. People lie when they pretend that they can do without poetry. The day they discover it, they realize how much they've missed it.

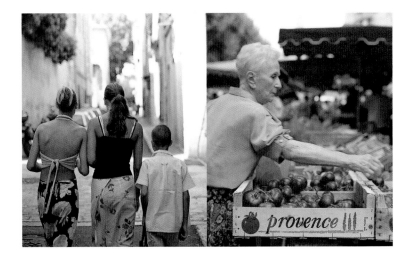

ABOVE AND RIGHT: FOR FRENCH WOMEN, COMFORTABLE DOESN'T NECESSARILY MEAN BAGGY; BODY-SKIMMING CLOTHES LOOK AND FEEL COOL FOR HOT DAYS.

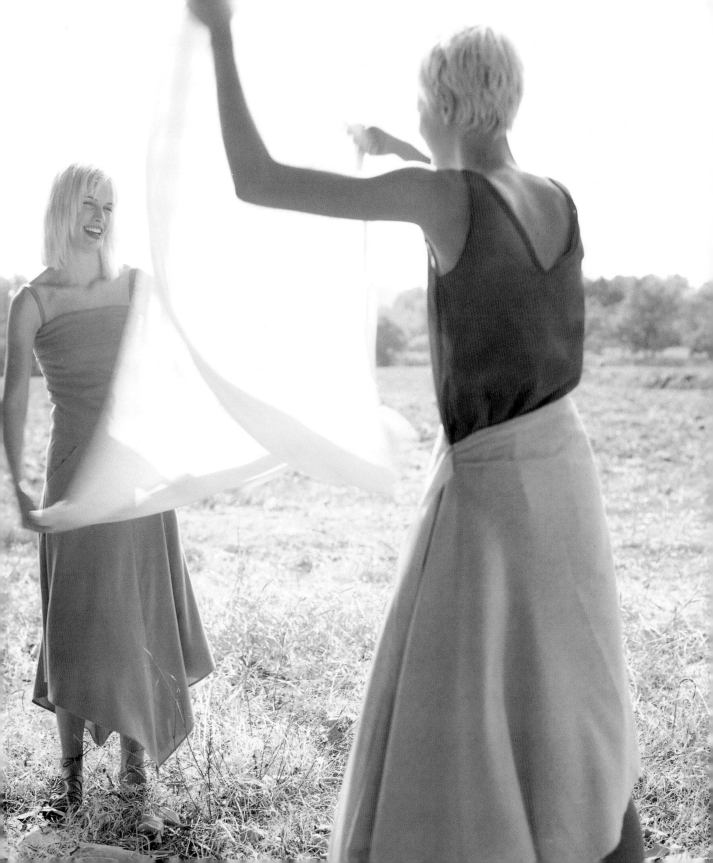

SUMMER MAKEUP

Summer makeup is almost an oxymoron. By the time August rolls around, most women I know have let their makeup routine slide (it's just too hot to apply foundation). The "barely there" look is the way to go; too much makeup can seem garish in the heat of August. At this time of the year, bronze-based color is a playful option—there's something both cheeky and charming about heightened color when the last of the summer fruit is at its peak.

THE BARELY-THERE SUMMER FACE

EYES Keep the eyes simple, using a light touch with a neutral, brownish tinged shadow. Apply the shadow over the lid and up to the brow bone, just enough to bring some extra definition. Use a light hand with the mascara, too (which can be very runny in the heat); a quick swipe over the lashes will suffice.

CHEEKS This is your chance to have some fun with a bronzer, one of the only times during the year when you can be extremely generous with your application. You can use a bronzer all over your face or rely on it to even out a tan. There is one simple trick to keep in mind: You want to focus on the parts of your face—such as the apples of the cheeks, top and sides of the forehead, bridge of the nose, tip of the chin—where the sun would naturally impart some color. Be careful not to use too dark a bronzer for your skin tone, otherwise your skin will just look dirty.

LIPS If you have a darker complexion, you can use a richer lip color to achieve this look. But whatever your coloring, stick with reddish browns on the lips. Apply a coat of a rich brownish lipstick over your lips and then use a lighter, but complementary, lip pencil just inside the lip line as a highlighter (it's easier to blend the lip pencil into the lipstick if applied second). This simple two-part process will give your lips more of a three-dimensional look, almost like a little free collagen injection, and your color will also last longer with the lip pencil.

NAILS Stick with a light and sheer nail color. A clean wash of pale champagne, with just a hint of shimmer, won't compete with your bronzed, summery face, but will finish off the look.

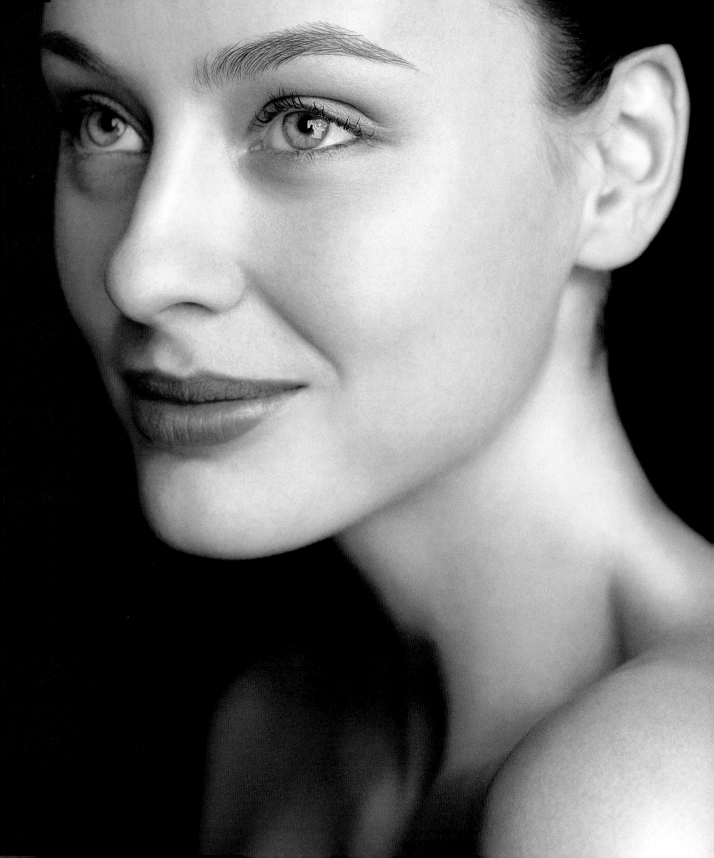

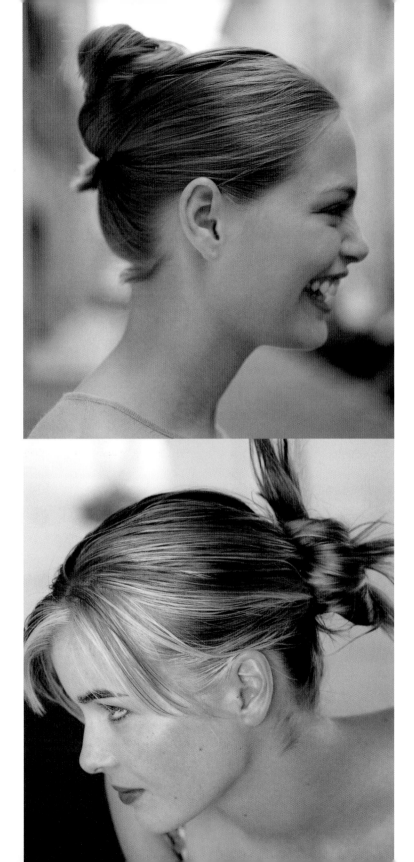

MAKE A MEDITERRANEAN-INSPIRED SALAD BY COMBINING THINLY SLICED PEARS, PROVOLONE, ARUGULA, FRESH MINT, AND BASIL. DRIZZLE AN OLIVE OIL AND CHAMPAGNE VINAIGRETTE ON TOP.

13

BUY GREAT NEW COLORFUL TOOTHBRUSHES FOR EVERYONE AT HOME.

14

THANK A FRIEND FOR INVITING YOU TO LUNCH, BUT DO NOT THANK HER FOR DINNER. INSTEAD, TELL HER HOW MUCH FUN YOU HAD, AND WHAT A GREAT PLEASURE IT WAS TO MEET THE OTHER GUESTS. A DINNER INVITATION DESERVES MORE THAN A SIMPLE THANK YOU.

15

SUMMER UPDO'S

Summer is action-packed. With the warm weather, you don't want to sit long in front of a mirror. You want to ease up on the fuss and be on the move. Putting your hair up will free you from worrying about having to be perfectly coiffed when you're spending more time outdoors or in humid weather.

If you know you'll be wearing your hair up rather than in a sleek, blown-out style, you will want to make some changes to your hair-care routine.

* Wash your hair with your regular shampoo, but use an extra-rich conditioner to plump up your hair shaft.
* Let your hair dry naturally. For even more bounce, towel it dry.
* Sweep your hair up into a bun or a half-ponytail. Don't waste time trying to coax each strand into place—the result would be too contrived.
* Once your hair is up, anchor your bun with big hairpins or a hair accessory— and let it be! For a casual, fresh look, let the ends fall free rather than tucking them in.
* For extra shine and texture, spritz on your favorite finishing product.
* If you really want to capture the playfulness of the summer and defy all the rules, use unexpected hair accessories such as pencils, twigs, flowers, earrings, or colorful strips of fabric.

Summer is about letting go and enjoying yourself, so give your hair permission to fall into place naturally. Let it bounce with the action: the sea breeze, the salty waves, the sound of music, the rhythm of the dance, and the swing of your tennis racquet.

APPLE-CIDER VINEGAR

If there's one thing that can simplify your beauty routine, it's a bottle of apple-cider vinegar. In France, women use it to clarify both their skin and hair. You can use it as a rinse after shampooing and conditioning to get rid of any residue left by styling products, or even as a shampoo itself. It will leave your hair shinier and healthier than you can imagine, especially if you rinse out the vinegar with ice-cold water. It's a jolt to the system, and the results are fantastic.

As a face cleanser, the apple-cider vinegar does many of the same things it does for the scalp and hair: stimulates blood flow, invigorates, and cleanses softly but thoroughly. Think of it as a wake-up tonic for your skin and hair, sort of the way you'd do a fast juice for your body. It's also great to take traveling, to counterbalance very hard water.

16

WASHING YOUR SKIN TOO OFTEN CAN MAKE IT DRY, ITCHY, OR EVEN OILY. **TRUST THE NATURAL CHEMISTRY OF YOUR SKIN** TO FIND ITS OWN BALANCE. TOO MUCH SCRUBBING IS COUNTERPRODUCTIVE.

17

RELIEVE HEAT-RELATED PUFFINESS IN YOUR FINGERS BY SOAKING YOUR HANDS FOR FIVE MINUTES IN COLD WATER MIXED WITH SEA SALT.

18

BUY FRESH SPICES AND THROW AWAY OLD ONES.

RELAXED HOSPITALITY

Provence is famous for its hospitality. During the summer, people come in droves from the North, seeking the sun, and often all the hotels are booked. So it is a tradition for the natives of Provence to keep their homes open to friends. They try to think of every possible way to put visitors at ease. I am no exception. For me, getting ready for overnight guests is something I love to do. But since I live in America, not in the South of France, my salons in the States are my homes. There, I try to treat my clients as I would if they came to see me in Aix.

Taking care of overnight guests who come to spend the weekend or the week with you is not unlike running a hair salon. Before guests arrive, you prepare their room and leave a stack of towels and a couple of terry-cloth robes. By the bed, you place a carafe of water with glasses, a scented candle, and maps and guidebooks to the area. Then you fill the house with flowers, either picked in your garden or bought at the local farmer's market. Nothing is "arranged," nothing is pretentious, nothing is blatantly expensive. When the decor is casual, everyone feels relaxed.

Each little thing you prepare for your guests in advance will increase their sense of well-being. Here is a list of small details that will make their stay in your house a truly unforgettable experience:

* **ALWAYS HAVE FLOWERS IN THEIR BEDROOM.** Or place blossoms or rose petals in a bowl of water in the bathroom.
* **SPRAY THEIR ROOM** with *essence de lavande,* spritzing sheets and inside drawers. The scent is clean and restful, yet never overwhelming.
* **IN THE BATHROOM,** leave a selection of bath gels, soaps, and lotions.

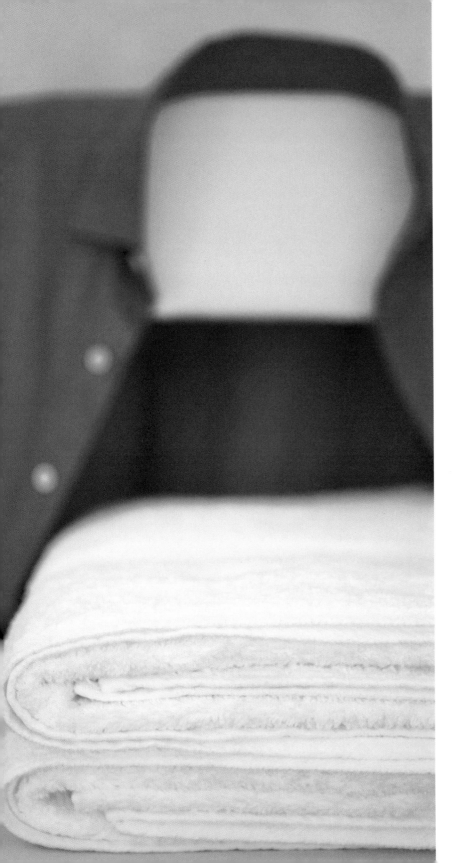

HOME SCENTS

There's an incredible hotel in St.-Paul-de-Vence, a little village that hovers high above the Riviera, called La Colombe d'Or. It has a gorgeous green pool, a heart-stopping view, priceless Picassos and Cézannes, and an unbelievable restaurant. Yet, the impression that really lingers is the way they spray lavender water on the sheets and pillowcases, making every night restful and oh so lightly scented.

I believe that every house should have a subtle yet distinctive fragrance signature. Bouquets of fresh flowers that provide visual as well as olfactory stimulation are my first choice: I am partial to big white Casablanca lilies in pitchers, full-blown roses in wide bowls, and strands of fragrant honeysuckle winding their way through a bunch of wildflowers, or planted in a windowbox.

Sprays in beautiful bottles are a fabulous alternative, and so are bags and sachets filled with scent that can be tucked away in the most unexpected places: in drawers and closets, in pockets, or even in the medicine cabinet, between the aspirin bottle and the shaving cream.

19

A STRAW-COLORED RUG ON
THE FLOOR MAKES ANY ROOM
FEEL LIKE SUMMER. A WOVEN
STRAW HANDBAG DOES THE
SAME THING FOR ALMOST ANY
OUTFIT.

20

RELAX BY READING BOOKS
ABOUT NATURE, HISTORY,
AND LOVE.

21

CARRY A LARGE SILK SCARF
WITH YOU TO COVER YOUR
SHOULDERS WHEN YOU GO IN
AN OVERLY AIR-CONDITIONED
RESTAURANT OR THEATER.

GIVING OUTDOOR PARTIES

For me, the sense of belonging to a family—whether a small group of relatives or an extended tribe—is the foundation of life. But a family is not just the people. It's also a collection of smells, sights, impressions, and memories. During the summer, children learn how to arrange flowers in a vase. How to pour juice from a jar. How to set a pretty table. How fruits taste when you pluck them from trees. How much fun it is to help with the dishes. And when it's time to say *good-bye*.

A great summer party is almost inevitably about the outdoors: I favor spur-of-the-moment, drag-the-tables-outside lunches and dinners, thrown together because a friend is passing through town, or a relative has a birthday, or simply because the day is so beautiful, the flowers in the garden so fragrant, and the moon so full. And I know that all these impromptu parties will be the source of great memories for my son Alexandre. What better opportunity for him to learn to get along with everyone and acquire an intimate appreciation of the good things in life.

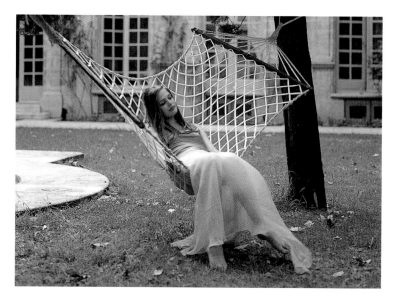

A SUMMER PARTY CHECKLIST

* INVITE PEOPLE WHO LOVE TO TALK and people who love to listen in equal numbers, if possible.

* WELCOME A FEW CRASHERS; they'll spice things up.

* COME UP WITH A THEME. It puts everyone in the spirit right off the bat.

* CONSIDER RENTING A SMALL TENT, one that accommodates about twenty people—the perfect number for an interesting party. Keep the flaps open to catch the breeze.

* HANG A HAMMOCK between two trees or place a bench in the shade.

* AN INVITATION builds anticipation and sets the mood. It doesn't have to be formal; a funny invitation is often best. Always specify what sort of dress is expected.

* THEN AGAIN, if the night is beautiful, pick up the phone and call some friends for an impromptu gathering. These can be the best parties of all.

* USE LOTS OF CANDLES in lanterns. Candlelight puts everyone in a romantic mood. The best summer party decorations are lots of pillows. When people sit on the floor, they instantly relax.

* MUSIC IS CRUCIAL. Consider live musicians or a deejay.

* PLAN A SIMPLE MENU, with the freshest ingredients. Unless you are a great chef, too much fussing makes food less tasteful.

* DON'T GO OVERBOARD on choices; focus on preparing a few great dishes rather than many so-so ones. The same goes for drinks: lemonade, rose champagne, and sparkling water are all you need.

* LIKE THE FOOD, THE FLOWERS should always be of the season. Pick them from your own garden, if possible—there's nothing more charming.

* ALWAYS HAVE PLENTY OF ICE, and plenty of shade.

RIGHT: PETANQUES, THE FRENCH VERSION OF BOCCI,
IS A VERY PROVENÇAL GAME. IT IS OFTEN PLAYED
IN THE MAIN SQUARES OF TOWNS AND VILLAGES.

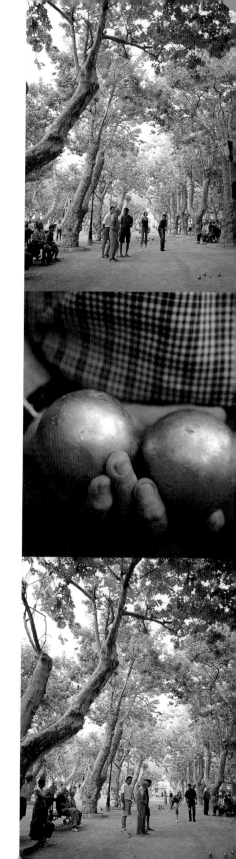

22

Go to Paris and become a woman.

—NAPOLEON

23

DON'T WEAR A SUN HAT WITH YOUR READING GLASSES. IT LOOKS FRUMPY. IF YOU LIKE TO READ OUTDOORS, INVEST IN A SMART PAIR OF PRESCRIPTION SUNGLASSES INSTEAD.

24

THIS MONTH AND NEXT IS THE **TIME TO EAT FIGS:** WASH THEM CAREFULLY AND CUT THEM IN HALF WITH A SHARP KNIFE. SERVE WITH THIN SHEETS OF PROSCIUTTO. DRINK CHAMPAGNE.

AN EASY SUMMER FEAST

The secret of a simple yet delicious buffet menu is to use the best seasonal ingredients, nothing exotic, nothing imported. Fresh local produce requires the least preparation.

To make your guests feel part of the family, and to encourage them to relax, ask them to help you set the food on the buffet table at the last minute. Send someone into the garden to find some herbs to decorate a platter. Give someone else the responsibility of chopping parsley. Put two people who don't know each other in charge of lighting the candles. Prompt your guests to get involved in the preparations. They'll feel like instant insiders and your party will take off right away. Don't forget the music—inside *and* out. Choose very lively, entertaining music, like Gipsy Kings or Santana.

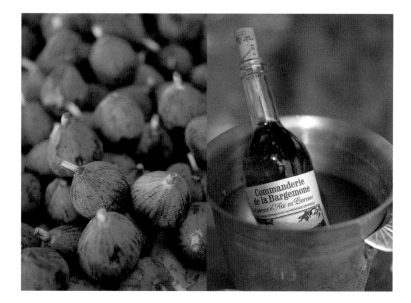

ABOVE: FIGS AND A ROSÉ WINE FROM PROVENCE ARE A LIGHT AND ORIGINAL TASTE COMBINATION FOR SUMMER.

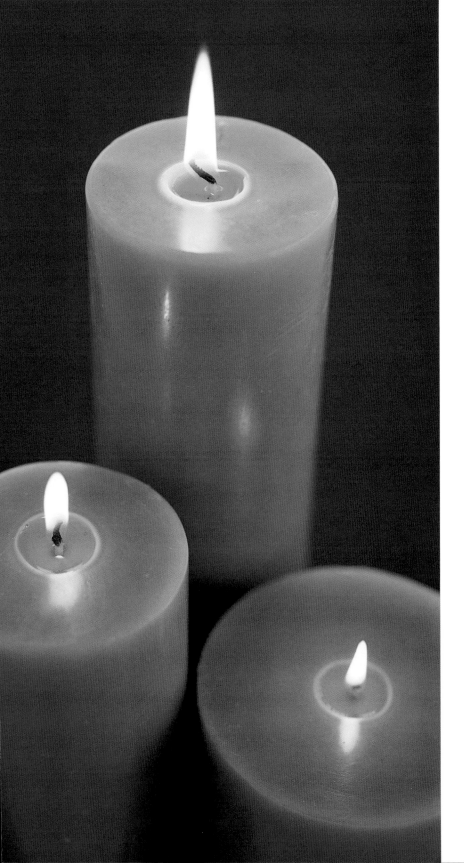

A CANDLELIGHT PRIMER

Candles add instant ambience: relaxing, slightly sexy. Set up a group to greet guests as they come through the front door.

✳ CLUSTERS OF SMALL, LOW CANDLES, or votives, are best on a table where you want people to be able to see each other.

✳ USE UNSCENTED CANDLES near where you'll be eating.

✳ TALL, THIN CANDLES are very formal; TALL, THICK CANDLES are wonderful in groups of differing sizes around a room.

✳ FLOAT CANDLES in wide glass vases or bowls; add flower blossoms or rose petals to the water.

✳ CITRONELLA CANDLES in small buckets or terra-cotta pots help to scare away bugs.

✳ I ALSO LOVE THE TORCHES you can stake in the ground. I use them to line pathways or to define the space around an outdoor party. They convey a sense of wildness and abandon.

✳ CANDELABRA are impossibly romantic.

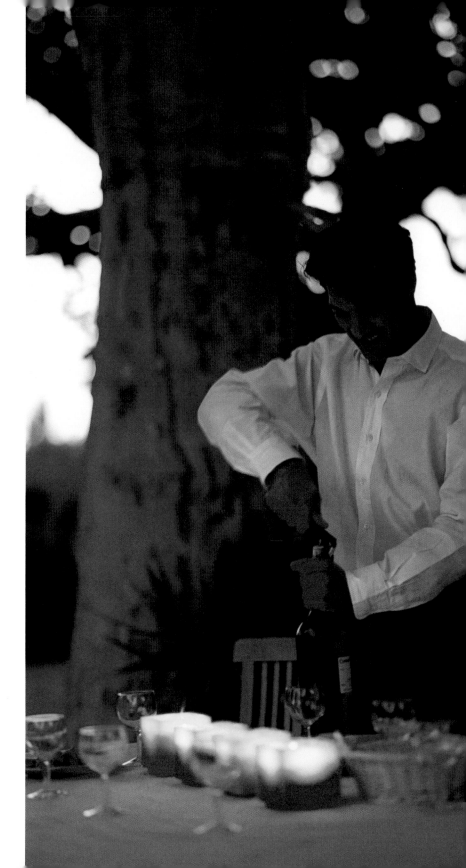

SUMMER FOOD

These dishes are colorful, fun to prepare, healthy, and festive.

∗ RASPBERRY ICED TEA, with fresh raspberries

∗ ROSÉ WINE served over ice

∗ SLICES OF RAW SALMON AND TUNA, marinated in olive oil, lemon, and parsley

∗ THIN SLICES OF TOASTED COUNTRY BREAD with tapenade, a black-olive-and-anchovy spread

∗ GRILLED SEA BASS with roasted tomatoes and fennel

∗ BOW-TIE PASTA SALAD with mozzarella, tomatoes, fresh basil, and crushed garlic

∗ TINY STEAMED POTATOES with butter, coarse sea salt, and lots of chopped parsley

∗ FRESH FIGS to eat with local goat cheese

∗ CHILLED BALLS OF WATER-MELON flavored with fresh lemon juice and mint leaves

THE PERFECT HOST

Prepare everything in advance, but don't fuss over your guests when they arrive. A mellow, serene host is a welcoming sight for harried travelers.

To help them catch their breath, set the example by being low-key. Go about your own business while they unpack at leisure. Treat them like family: Watch over them, give them keys, explain about the alarm if need be, show them how to use the phone, the dishwasher, the espresso maker, and make sure they have enough hangers for their clothes, but don't try to organize their life or act as their social director.

Make it clear that they don't have to follow your schedule, and that you are not going to wait for them to decide what they want to do. Still, take the time to advise them on what to see, so that they don't miss the most interesting natural sights and historical landmarks in the area. And of course, tell them about the best local restaurants and which house specialties to order.

When you visit a place, tasting local food deepens your experience of it. When my American or European friends come to my place in Provence, I like to have something for them to eat prepared in advance, so they can help themselves at their convenience. I spend the day before their arrival shopping for the healthiest organic food and the most delicious specialties I can find at local markets.

It's so much fun, sometimes I wonder if having overnight guests is not a pretext for me to sample all the best gourmet products, from the finest breakfast jams and pastries to the rarest liqueurs.

Adapt these suggestions to your particular locale and local produce:

* **MAKE GREAT PITCHERS OF ICED HERB TEA** by pouring boiling water directly on fresh mint leaves and allowing it to cool.
* **MAKE FRESH LEMONADE,** called *citron pressé,* by stirring together lemon juice, ice, water, and sugar.

LISTEN TO VIVALDI IN THE MORNING WHILE YOU STRETCH. 25

FLAVOR HOMEMADE ICE CREAM WITH LAVENDER TEA AND HONEY. IT'S A PROVENÇAL SPECIALTY. 26

SMILE WHEN PICKING UP THE PHONE. THE CALLER WILL HEAR IT IN YOUR VOICE. 27

28 NEVER INTERRUPT WHEN YOU ARE BEING FLATTERED.

29

I base most of my fashion taste on what doesn't itch.

—GILDA RADNER

30 BEFORE RETIRING TO BED, **SLATHER YOUR FEET** IN A RICH MOISTURIZING CREAM AND SLIP ON A PAIR OF LIGHT COTTON SOCKS.

31 **GO BACK-TO-SCHOOL SHOPPING** WITH A NIECE OR FRIEND'S DAUGHTER AND SPLURGE ON AN OUTFIT FOR HER.

---

* **SET OUT BIG TRAYS OF CRUDITÉS:** tiny raw artichokes, cauliflower florets, cucumbers, tomatoes, radishes, onions, peppers, haricots verts, hard-boiled eggs accompanied with soft butter and salt, olive oil, or an aïoli, a garlicky homemade mayonnaise.

* **PURCHASE BREAD** from the oldest bakery in town and an assortment of jams from a farm stand.

* **GET AN ASSORTMENT OF PÂTÉS AND TERRINES** from the farmer down the road.

* **BUY A HUGE SELECTION**—as many as fifty—different local cheeses from the market (they keep for a long time, a month at least).

* **MAKE A PLATTER OF TOMATO SCRAMBLED EGGS,** a Provençal specialty called *pipérade,* using fresh tomato sauce.

* **PURCHASE LOCAL ORGANIC WINE.**

I learned to be a good host from watching my friends Gil Dez, Daniel Jouve, and Charles Montemarco run the Villa Gallici hotel in Aix-en-Provence. Perched on a hill just outside the center of town on what used to be an orchard, this small, exclusive hotel has a huge pool and an enormous terrace surrounded by hundred-year-old plane trees, olive trees, almond trees, and bougainvillea vines. A dream retreat, it is as comfortable and luxurious indoors as it is outdoors. I go there for lunch and then I take a nap by the pool, and no one ever makes me feel guilty for dozing till four in the afternoon.

In the same way, when I see one of my guests asleep in the hammock, or taking a snooze under a tree with a book over his face, I know that I have been the perfect host.

RIGHT: RAW RADISHES DIPPED IN COARSE SEA SALT ARE TRADITIONAL COCKTAIL FARE IN FRANCE.

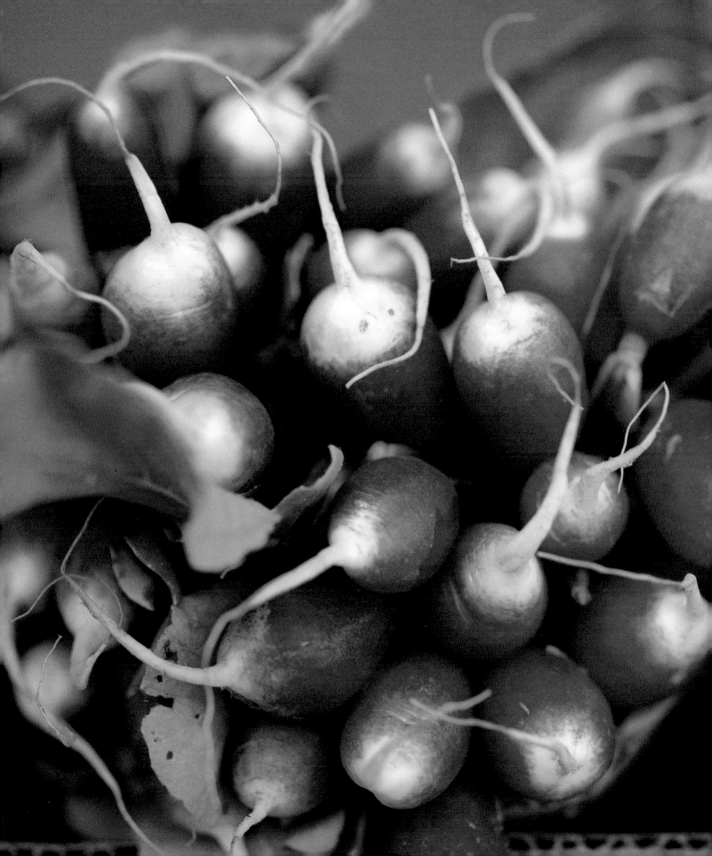

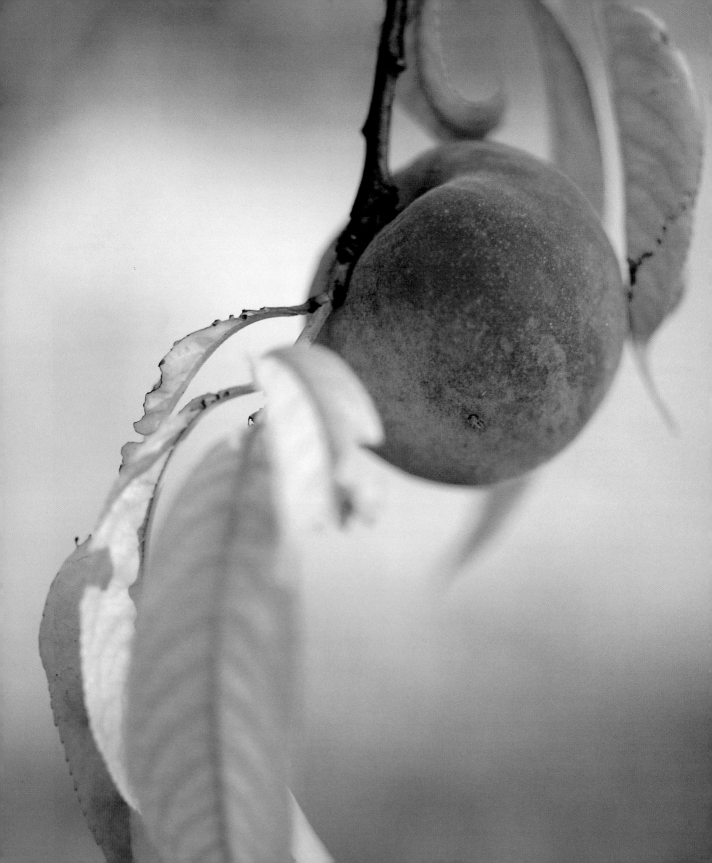

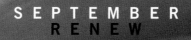

SEPTEMBER
RENEW

Does fashion matter? Only if you are out of it.

—KIM CAMPBELL

1

2

CELEBRATE THE BEGINNING OF FALL: **BUY A NEW LIPSTICK** IN A DEEP AND MELLOW SHADE OF RED.

3

VARY YOUR EXERCISE ROUTINE: TRY BIKE RIDING IF YOU USUALLY RUN, OR SIGN UP FOR A BALLROOM DANCING CLASS INSTEAD OF AEROBICS.

It's September, at long last! For most of us, it is like New Year's all over again: We want new clothes, new makeup, a new bag, a new hairstyle. We are back at the gym. It's the beginning of a new school year and we're all eager to learn what's on the horizon, to assimilate the latest directions in fashion and beauty, see the new films, try the new restaurants. The leisurely pace of the summer is forgotten as we once again pack our schedules with appointments and events. Remaining stylish takes a bit more effort, a bit more finesse.

In September in my salons, clients discuss the fads of the season. They have devoured the September fashion magazines through and through and want to know what I think of the new trends. Should hems go up or down? Is green done and orange au courant? I try to be diplomatic in my answers, but basically, I am against trends. The shows in Milan, Paris, London,

RIGHT: A SIMPLE KNIT TANK UNDER A TAILORED JACKET IS THE PERFECT WAY TO EDGE BACK INTO FALL.

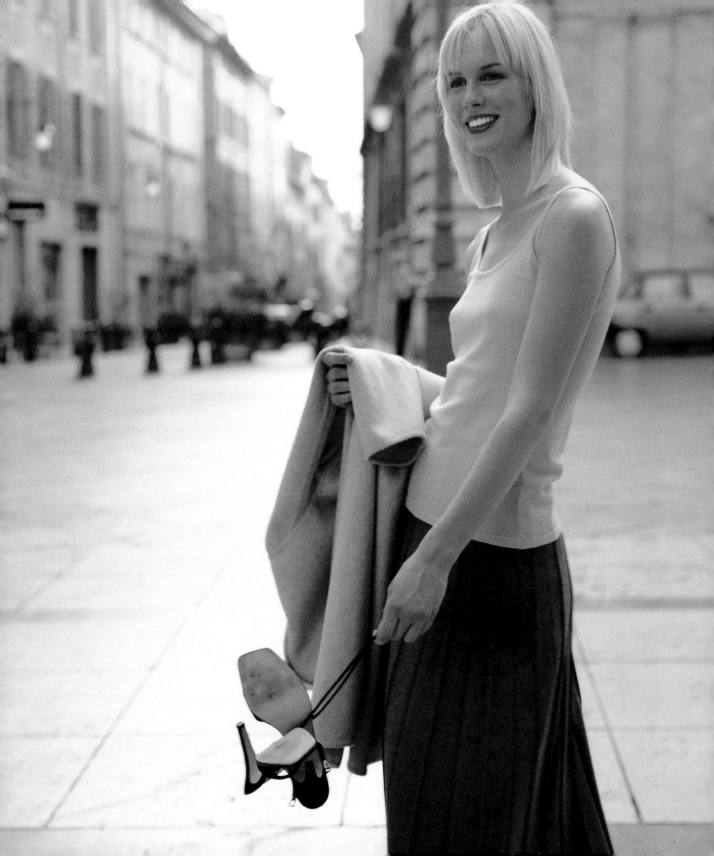

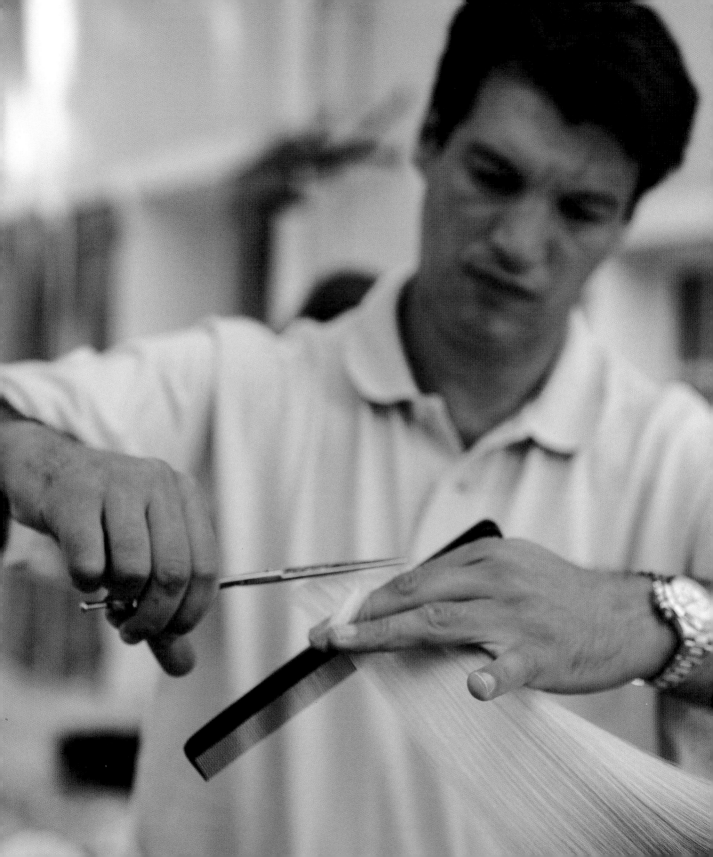

and New York are performance pieces designed to create a buzz for the designer. As far as I am concerned, "trendy" is "passé" the minute it hits the streets, and "cool" is un-cool on anyone out of high school. Trends are great entertainment, but are essentially worthless when it comes to real life.

Don't get me wrong, though: Avoiding trends does not mean ignoring fashion. To the contrary, I am always telling my clients how to update their look, how to stay current, in the know. There is nothing worse than someone who is stuck in time, with clothes, hair, and makeup that are even slightly outmoded.

A fresh and modern look is easy to achieve as long as you realize that there is no such a thing as permanent perfection. Even after you've found a look, or an attitude that is comfortable to you, you'll need to hone it, refine it, making minor adjustments to your hair, makeup, and wardrobe every season—even day to day. It could be something as simple as replacing your neutral brown handbag with a dark green or burgundy one, picking a deeper, more opaque lip color, or changing your neckline from a jewelneck to a squared-off boatneck under a suit, to more radical changes to hair color or length. The nature of the change is less important than the constant re-evaluation.

The worst mistake a woman can make is trying to look the same way every day. A French proverb illustrates this point: *Tous les jours se suivent mais ne se ressemblent pas:* "No day is exactly like the one it follows." In other words, what looks beautiful on you today will not necessarily look beautiful on you tomorrow. You may be tired. Or in better shape. Or in love.

So don't try to duplicate yesterday's look. Forget last week's hairdo. Shelve last month's great idea. Retire last season's color scheme.

Be new today. It works every time.

REORGANIZE YOUR CLOSET WITH FALL AND WINTER ACCESSORIES. **4**

TRADE IN YOUR BRIGHT SUMMER NAIL POLISH FOR SOMETHING MORE SOPHISTICATED, LIKE BORDEAUX, PINOT NOIR, ZINFANDEL, OR BURGUNDY—THE COLORS OF FULL-BODIED RED WINES. **5**

DONATE ALL THOSE SUMMER BEST-SELLERS YOU WON'T REREAD TO A NURSING HOME OR A HOSPITAL. **6**

LEFT: EVEN IF YOU'RE NOT READY FOR A MAJOR CHANGE, A GOOD TRIM WILL GIVE YOU A CLEAN LOOK FOR THE NEW SEASON.

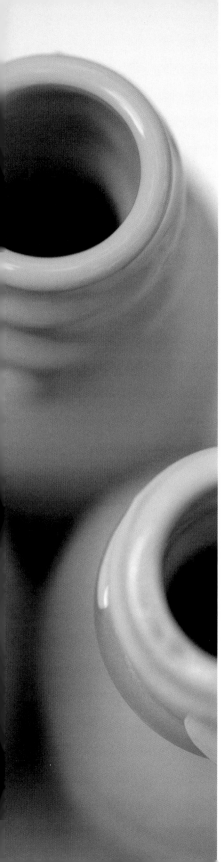

RENEW YOUR MAKEUP ROUTINE

Remember the reason you put makeup on: It's to make you look better, not to make you look as if you've got great makeup on. Makeup should be invisible when applied, otherwise it will age you. The following three rules will take years off your face.

BEAUTY RULE #1

Concealer, judiciously placed, can do more for you than any other product.

BEAUTY RULE #2

There should be no distinct lines—on lips, on lids, anywhere—visible on your face.

BEAUTY RULE #3

Never put powder under the eyes, it will highlight wrinkles that were otherwise invisible to the naked eye.

FOUNDATION If you don't need foundation, by all means, skip it. That said, if you feel naked bare-faced, pick a formula that seems to disappear on your skin. Healthy-looking skin, rather than a mask of foundation, is what you should see.

* **WHETHER YOU USE A LIQUID,** powder, stick, cream, or a tinted-moisturizer foundation formula, apply it before you put on concealer. Then it's obvious what you still need to cover up.
* **MATCH FOUNDATION** to the skin on your face, not your arm, not the back of your hand. The skin at your jawline is a good spot to test, as you want it to blend with the skin on your neck as well.
* **APPLY FOUNDATION WITH A LIGHT HAND**—a little goes a long way. You can always add more if you need to.

* **LET FRECKLES SHOW THROUGH.** They're so charming.
* **DON'T USE FOUNDATION** to try to cover dark circles or blemishes. That's what concealer is designed to do.
* **NEVER USE FOUNDATION AS A WAY** of darkening your skin tone. The finish will be unnatural, no matter what you do. Bronzing gels or powders are a much better way to achieve this. Remember, however, if you use any sort of bronzer, your neck must match your face.

CONCEALER Concealer can change your look incredibly, and up your confidence level in the bargain. Just dab a bit on anything you're not so happy with. But do use it sparingly, as most concealers have very concentrated pigment.

* **LIKE FOUNDATION,** concealer should match your skin tone as closely as possible. If in doubt, err on the lighter side, as the things you're concealing (under-eye circles, blemishes, uneven pigment) tend to be darker than your skin tone. Just don't go too light or you risk highlighting your imperfections.
* **ALWAYS APPLY CONCEALER WITH A BRUSH.** It leaves a much more natural finish on the skin than using a finger, because it deposits the color exactly where you want it. Many of my makeup artists dab the brush in the concealer, then stroke the brush on their palms, to get rid of any excess. Use as little pigment as you can, and place it only where you need it. To conceal under-eye circles, brush the concealer into the shadow caused by the puffiness, never on the puffiness (which would accent the circle).
* **ONCE YOU'VE BRUSHED ON THE CONCEALER,** pat to blend. Never, ever rub, as that just moves the concealer away from where you want it. Think of tapping it, even pressing it into your skin. You'll think it isn't going to blend, then, tap, tap, tap, and suddenly it has disappeared, along with your blemishes or blotches.
* **USE A VELVETY PUFF** to press powder very lightly onto the spot you've just concealed, to help the concealer stay in place.

PAINT JUST ONE WALL IN YOUR BEDROOM IN A REALLY GREAT COLOR SUCH AS RUSSET, OCHER, OR VENETIAN RED. RED MAKES YOU LOOK MORE BEAUTIFUL WHEN YOU WAKE UP.

7

SIGN UP FOR PUBLIC-SPEAKING LESSONS: "PROPER WORDS IN PROPER PLACES MAKE THE TRUE DEFINITION OF A STYLE," SAID JONATHAN SWIFT.

8

PROLONG YOUR TAN WITH A SELF-TANNING TREATMENT.

9

10

GO THOUGH YOUR WALLET,
REMOVING EVERYTHING
THAT'S NOT ESSENTIAL.
UPDATE ANY PHOTOGRAPHS
YOU CARRY AROUND
WITH YOU.

11

*Beauty can pierce
one like pain.*
—THOMAS MANN

12

MEDITATE. FIVE MINUTES
A DAY IS ALL YOU NEED TO
INCREASE YOUR SELF-ESTEEM
AND SELF-CONFIDENCE.

POWDER Most women can benefit from powder. It both sets your makeup to keep it looking fresh and true, and absorbs excess oil to keep shine in check. Remember, however, that a bit of a glow is definitely good; you might need powder only in the t-zone, rather than all over your face.

* **CONSIDER TRANSLUCENT POWDER** with a bit of yellow in it, to warm the skin tone.
* **TO REALLY KEEP MAKEUP IN PLACE,** roll on powder with a puff using just a little pressure. Then, brush off excess with a soft brush.
* **TOO MUCH POWDER** leaves a very matte, sometimes crepe-y finish. Not a good look. To apply just the right amount of powder, always tap puff or blow on brush to remove excess before applying to skin.
* **MULTIPLE LAYERS OF PRESSED POWDER** applied throughout the day can give your makeup a cakey look, so avoid constant touch-ups. If you have oily skin, blot with a tissue first to remove excess oil.
* **POWDERING YOUR FACE IN PUBLIC** is aging, tacky—just wrong.

BLUSH When blush is applied correctly you look like you've got healthy color in your cheeks, and that's all. Never use blush to contour—contouring is for professionals, on photo shoots. It looks crazy in real life. Always err on the side of too little.

* **PLAY WITH BLUSH SHADES** to determine what works with your skin tone. A plum-colored blush can look pink on the skin. So can a red one. You have to experiment.
* **SMILE.** The apple of your cheek is where the blush goes. A little pink blush on the apple of the cheeks makes almost anyone look instantly brighter, younger.
* **CREAM BLUSH** leaves a very appealing, dewy finish. Apply it with your fingers or a little sponge and blend well.
* **POWDER BLUSH** goes on more translucent, so it's a little more foolproof.

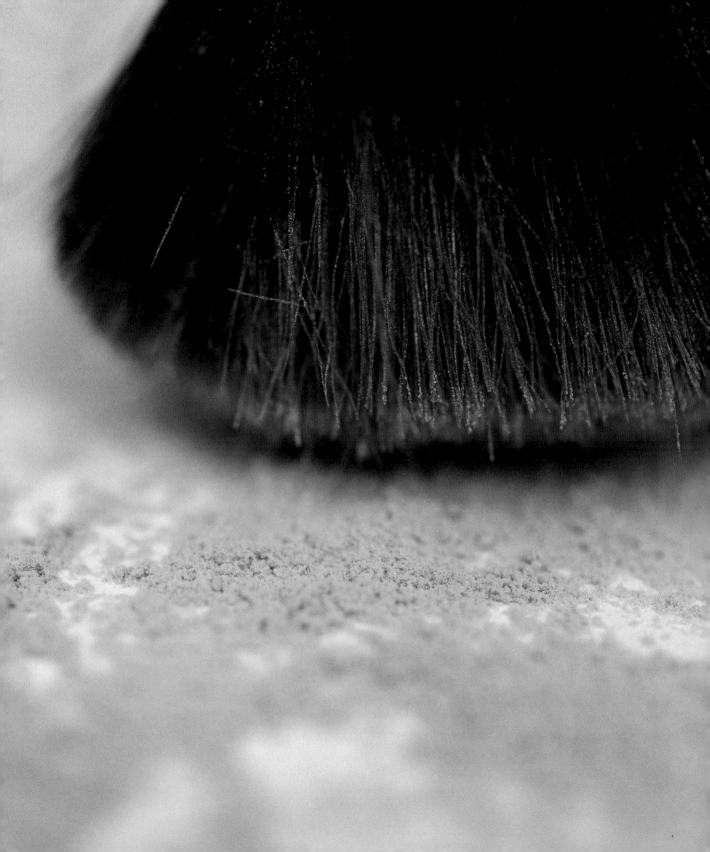

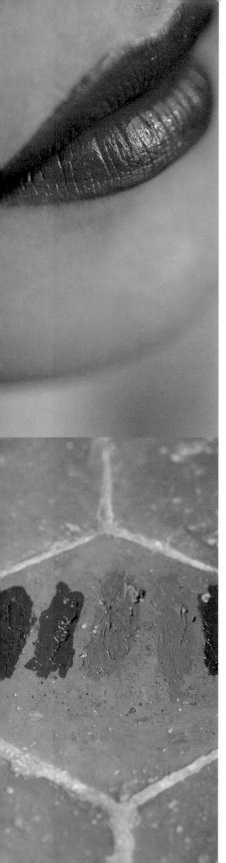

* **TO MAKE BLUSH REALLY POP** (subtly, of course), apply two colors: a neutral brown-based tone on first, with a pink on top.
* **IF YOU'RE TRYING TO DARKEN YOUR SKIN TONE,** use a big brush to apply a bronze-colored blush or bronzing powder to cheeks, plus a hint on the forehead, chin, and nose. Overdoing it looks artificial. Remember, pale skin can be beautiful, too.
* **BLEND, BLEND, BLEND.**
* **IF YOU HAVE A LONG OR VERY THIN FACE,** apply blush with horizontal strokes and keep it away from the sides of your face.

LIPSTICK, GLOSS, AND STAINS Find one you absolutely love: Color, texture, smell, even the package should be a pleasure. Except for really major occasions, I like lips to look as natural as possible. Very intense shades and very thick, shiny gloss are hard to maintain throughout the day, and why would you want to? The glossier a formula, the more quickly it disappears. The more matte, the longer lasting. Lipstick, in the absence of any other makeup, can overwhelm your face. Use a sheer gloss if lips are all you're going to do.

* **SIMILARLY, ALWAYS BALANCE STRONGER LIP COLOR:** You'll want mascara, for instance, if you've got lipstick with real color or texture to it. Too much color or texture, without other makeup to balance it, can look cheap.
* **BROWNS, PLUMS, BURGUNDIES, PINKS,** and even some subtle red shades can all be fairly neutral. It depends on the formula, and, as always, you just have to keep trying different ones until you hit the jackpot: a great, natural-looking lip color that adds color to your face without adding the look of makeup with a capital M.
* **A REALLY MATTE LIP** is very aging.
* **A REALLY GLOSSY LIP** can look teeny-bopper-ish.

* **SHEER STAINS** are very natural-looking and long-lasting. Wear them with a bit of gloss on top to add shine and moisture.
* **LONG-LASTING LIPSTICKS** can create a false sense of security. They may last better in one spot than in another, and they're harder to reapply, as you need to take the first coat off (sometimes with remover) before you start again. If you do choose this formulation, use a neutral shade that's not terribly strong, so it's not as blotchy when it wears off.

LIP LINER Visible lip liner is one of the worst makeup faux pas there is. I'd rather see someone with shoes that didn't match. If you need lip liner (not everyone does, you know: Unless you're worried about your lipstick bleeding or fading, you probably don't), use a shade that blends so well with your natural color it becomes invisible. And forget about using it to draw in larger lips: If you've got really thin lips, use pencil all over the entire lip, rather than just a line. The more intense shade that you get from the all-over pencil will make your lips look bigger. In general, look for the right lip color to set off your lips, rather than trying to draw them on.

EYES: LINER, SHADOW, MASCARA Eyes are perhaps the most over-made-up part of most women's faces. For day, you're really trying to enhance your eyes, not make a dramatic statement.

* **SHEER, NEUTRAL SHADOWS**—taupe, beige, pale pale banana yellow, mushroom—flatter your eyes, yet keep the focus on you rather than your eye makeup.
* **DEPENDING ON YOUR PERSONALITY,** however, bright shades can work, as long as they're applied in a sheer way, a wash of color over the lid, like a watercolor. Experiment with stronger colors if you like them, and always use a brush, for that sheer wash effect.

READ THE LATEST BEST-SELLING BIOGRAPHY. EVERYONE WILL BE TALKING ABOUT IT THIS FALL. — 13

RUB FINISHING CREAM IN YOUR HAND BEFORE APPLYING TO YOUR HAIR; FINISHING CREAMS MAKE GREAT HAND SOFTENERS. A LITTLE GOES A LONG WAY, SO BE CONSERVATIVE AND REPEAT IF NEEDED. — 14

RETIRE YOUR COLORFUL T-SHIRTS UNTIL NEXT SUMMER. — 15

16 IF YOU LET YOUR BROW GO A LITTLE BIT DURING THE SUMMER, NOW IS THE TIME TO CLEAN IT UP AND REMOVE ANY EXTRANEOUS HAIR.

17 **SEND FOR THE FALL LECTURE SCHEDULE** FROM A LOCAL LIBRARY OR MUSEUM.

18 DON'T FORGET TO **MOISTURIZE YOUR ELBOWS** AS MUCH AS YOU DO YOUR HANDS.

* **TECHNIQUES THAT INVOLVE ELABORATE** eye-shadow-placement strategies (i.e., beige on the lid, brown at the crease, burgundy at the corners) are not modern and take more time than they're worth.

* **CREAM EYE SHADOW** can be too thick and look scaly on your lids, so be careful if you choose a cream formula. Powders are easier and can generally be applied more sheer.

* **UNLESS YOU'RE A PROFESSIONAL** makeup artist, liquid eyeliner is usually a bad idea. It's hard to apply and looks awful when done incorrectly.

* **NEVER PUT EYELINER** all the way around the eye. It's aging, no matter how old you are. If you want a little liner under the eye, use a very, very small amount, just under the outer corner of the eye, and always smudge the line and blend thoroughly.

* **AFTER USING AN EYE PENCIL,** smudge the line, then run a little shadow over it, to set it. It'll last much longer.

* **IF YOU PUT ON LINER** after putting on your mascara, you'll probably use less.

* **ALWAYS TAKE A MINUTE** to clean up liner—and any mascara smudges—with a Q-tip. Q-tips are right up there with the greatest makeup tools ever.

* **AN EYE SHADOW BASE,** extra step though it is, will make your shadow last longer. So will patting on a little translucent powder (using a puff rolled over your finger) to set the shadow.

* **MASCARA SHOULD BE** black or brown-black, period. Your eyelashes are not circus tents, so don't paint them green, red, or cobalt.

* **MASCARA SHOULD MAKE** your lashes look great, not look like they've got mascara on them. That fringe-of-black-needles look is really awful, as are globs and blobs. Use a comb, brush, tissue paper, or even your finger to thin out mascara once it's on your lashes.

CHIC DAYTIME MAKEUP

This is a very neat and polished look that will complement the crisp excitement of the fall season. It's natural and understated, so it won't overpower your face, and it is appropriate for just about any professional setting. Select neutral rose colors if your skin has pinkish undertones or your hair is fair. For skin with yellow undertones, lean more toward neutral browns and grays.

EYES Since this face conveys a clean, put-together look, a well-groomed brow is important. After you've finished grooming your brow, fill it in with a brow pencil that closely matches your brow color. Then, with a muted gray, rich brown, or classic navy pencil, draw a smooth line across your upper lid, following the lash line. Choose a shadow in a pale neutral color with a slight shimmer and with a brush, sweep the color across your lid, but not all the way to the brow bone. Blend the shadow and pencil carefully together so that the transition between the two is seamless. Finish the look with one coat of black mascara.

CHEEKS Pick a natural-colored blush in rose or brown and sweep it over the cheekbones, blending well to soften the color for a clean look.

LIPS Don't overpower this look with a strong lipstick color; go for a subtle rose earthy or neutral red in a cream formula or a slightly brighter, richer cranberry or plum in a sheer formula. The color should look fresh, warm, and classic.

NAILS Keep your nails short at this busy time of year. For polish, choose a pale champagne color, light rosy brown, or a richer neutral brown to complete this look.

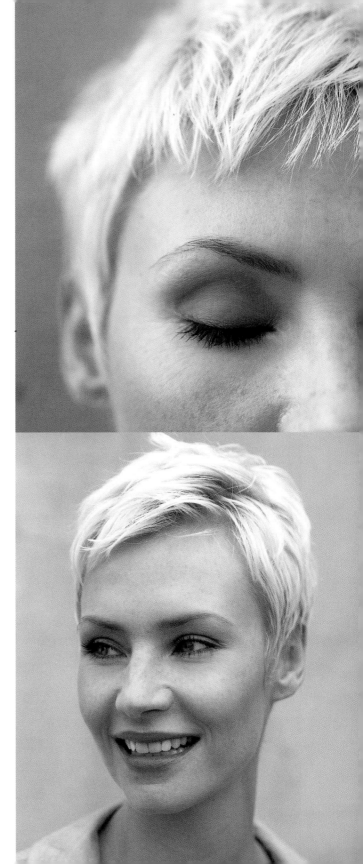

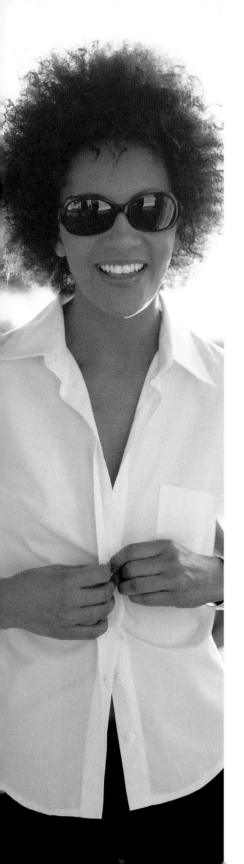

RENEWING YOUR WARDROBE

At this time of the year, it's only natural that you'd want to overhaul your closet completely, but beware of succumbing to trends. Even the chicest designer fashions, when they are taken up by everyone, stop being unique. And, with so many manufacturers now knocking off haute couture looks at reasonable prices, the best clothes and the greatest styles lose their originality and become stereotyped well before the end of the season.

On the other hand, it's essential to keep your look modern and fresh, not fixed in a moment in time. This shows insecurity, or, worse, ignorance. Some items, like a crisp white shirt or cashmere cardigan, are timeless, but even they can look tired paired with last year's skirt or the wrong trousers.

What is important when shopping is to combine the best of everything. Get a pair of loafers here, a dress there, a sweater somewhere else, a shirt at yet another address. In other words, you have to be your own stylist when you shop. You have to tell yourself that you are dressing a client, and that client is you! It requires becoming somewhat detached from your vanity. Focus on finding what works for you.

It's also a good idea to befriend boutique owners and get their advice as you stand in front of the mirror. Since their professional pride depends on your looking great, they are more likely to be straightforward and honest with their comments. Always take the remarks of mothers, girlfriends, and eager sales associates, however, with a grain of salt.

To be truly stylish, the best approach of all is to come up with fresh new ideas—on your own. This doesn't mean affecting an eccentrically eclectic mix of styles, but rather synthesizing what's available together with what's in your closet for a distinctive—and unique—look of your own.

LEFT AND RIGHT: NEUTRAL COLORS AND SEASONLESS FABRICS
CREATE A FABULOUS *PASSE-PARTOUT* (GO ANYWHERE) LOOK.

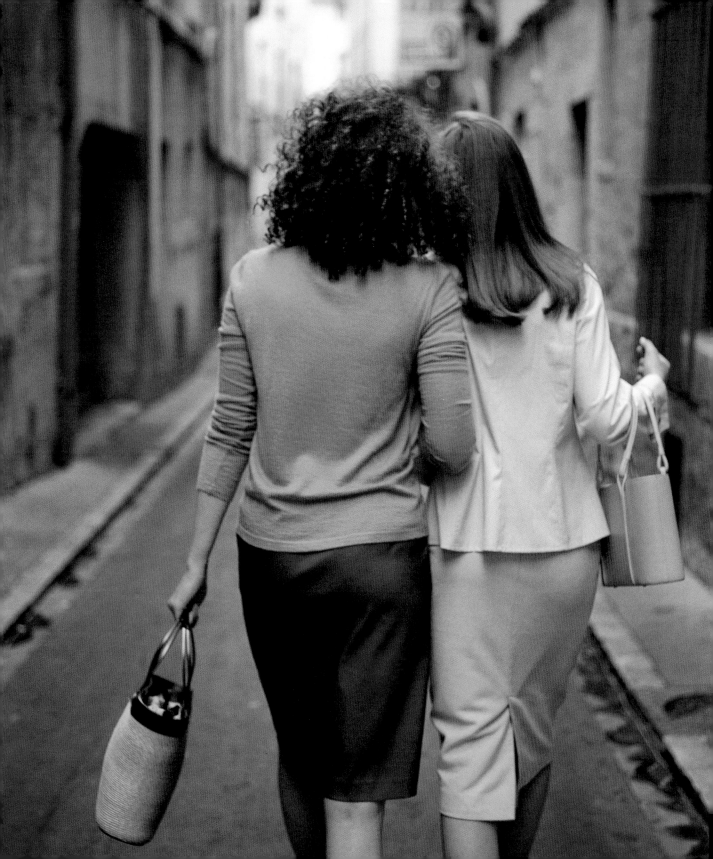

19 SAVE ON TAXI CABS IF YOU MUST, BUT **ALWAYS BUY THE BEST SHOES YOU CAN AFFORD.**

20 FIND SOMEONE IN YOUR NEIGHBORHOOD WHO CAN DO EXCELLENT ALTERATIONS. READY-TO-WEAR CLOTHES ARE LIKE HAIRCUTS: THEY USUALLY NEED ADJUSTMENTS.

21 **PUT AWAY YOUR COWBOY BOOTS.** NO ONE—NOT EVEN A REAL COWBOY—CAN PULL OFF A SOPHISTICATED URBAN WESTERN LOOK.

* **MAKE A COLLAGE OR FOLDER** of your favorite looks from the fall fashion issues, and take it along when you shop to help you define your own personal direction.
* **BEGIN BY SELECTING COLORS, NOT LABELS.** Create your own color palette from the clothes that have attracted your eye in fashion magazines.
* **WITH EACH OUTFIT, PICK ONE ACCESSORY TO CRYSTALLIZE THE LOOK.** Add an idiosyncratic touch: Buy a great belt. Or a fabulous bag. Or a new pair of glasses. Or the most amazing boots. All you need is one unique item, and your color-coordinated wardrobe will have a look of its own.

Shop for clothes the way you shop for antiques, one thing at a time, without rushing. Buy no more than two items from any one designer and never ever dress from head to toe in a single label. When you put on a designer outfit you become a walking billboard for his or her style—not your own.

That said, it can certainly be worth investing in a few flawlessly constructed pieces to anchor your wardrobe. Build on this foundation with less expensive or trendier (and more disposable) items. Finish with something distinctive and personal that shows your confidence in your own taste.

* **START WITH ONE ITEM,** usually something to wear on the bottom. Let's say you buy a flawless pair of pants from a prestigious designer.
* **ORDER A TOP,** maybe a white shirt, from your favorite catalog.
* **ADD SOME ARTISTIC JEWELRY** from a downtown boutique.

Suddenly you look like a million dollars. What could be easier!

RIGHT: MAGAZINES ARE A GOOD SOURCE OF INSPIRATION FOR BUILDING YOUR WARDROBE, BUT DON'T TAKE THEM AS GOSPEL. AN ARTFUL MIX OF PIECES IS MORE STYLISH THAN A HEAD-TO-TOE DESIGNER LOOK.

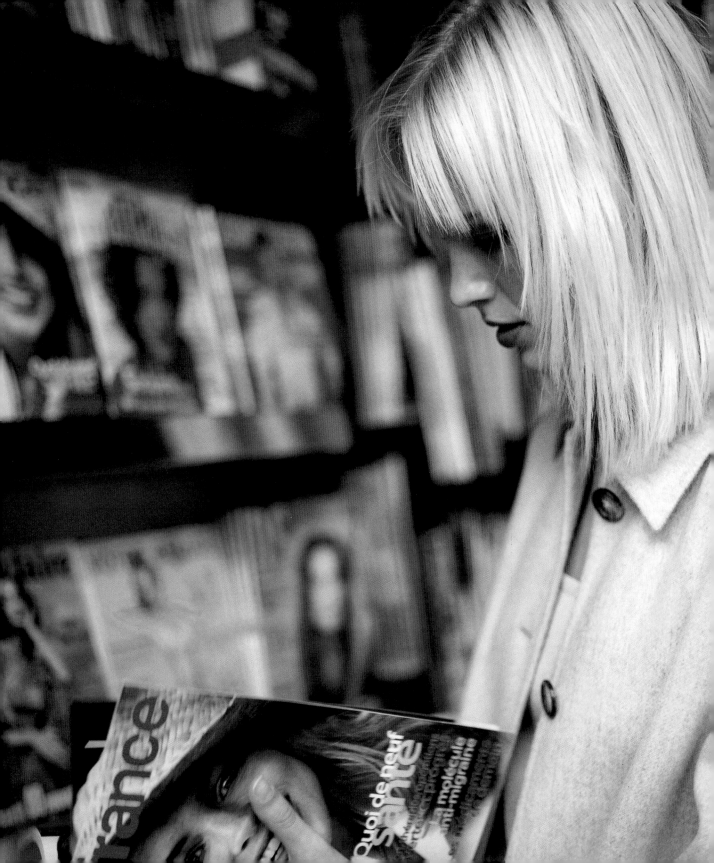

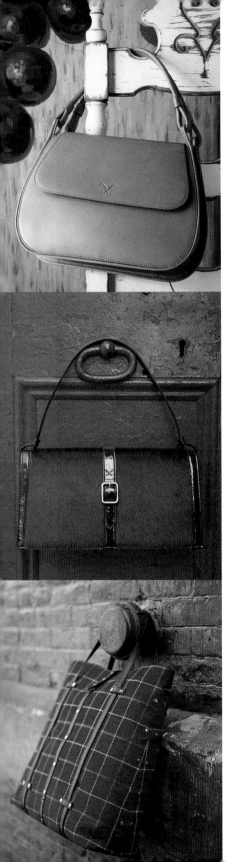

GREAT BAGS

Many clients are eager to have me pick out the right bag for them as the final touch to complete their individual style. The thing is, the right bag for one person can be completely wrong for another. Choosing a bag, that workhorse of an accessory, is not unlike deciding what sort of haircut to get; lifestyle is very important. Consider the following:

* **WHAT IS THE INTENDED PURPOSE OF THE BAG?** Is it just for going out? Is it the only bag you'll carry, or do you have several? Does it need to go with everything? What are you going to be carrying—Is it big enough for your cell phone? That bottle of water you take everywhere? Your gym clothes?

* **WHAT KIND OF IMAGE DO YOU WANT TO PROJECT?** Something very structured in basic black, navy, or brown, says "I'm conservative," while a bag with embroidery, buttons, or even appliqués says "I'm playful."

* **LEATHER, SUEDE, FUR,** and even nylon are perfect in the fall or winter.

* **TINY BAGS ARE CUTE,** but make sure you don't get one so small you can't fit essentials into it. Do you need glasses? Wallet? Makeup? Comb? Cell phone? Tiny bags should never bulge.

* **REALLY BIG BAGS CAN POSE PROBLEMS:** The larger they are, the more likely you are to throw things in that aren't essential. You end up carrying pounds of stuff around, which can eventually strain your back, not to mention the nuisance you go through looking for things that get lost in the jumble. Save big bags for weekend jaunts or air travel carry-ons.

* **WHAT SHAPES DO YOU LOVE?** Watch other people, especially women with a style similar to yours, to see what shapes look best out in the real world.

* **ARE YOUR CLOTHES STRUCTURED AND TAILORED?** Then a sturdier construction and geometrical shape would suit you. If your clothes are looser and more relaxed, a soft bag in a more organic shape would be right for you.

* **A GREAT BAG PROJECTS A SENSE OF ATTITUDE;** the shape, the material it's made out of, and the trim all contribute to it.

* **IF A BAG MAKES YOU SMILE, BUY IT.**

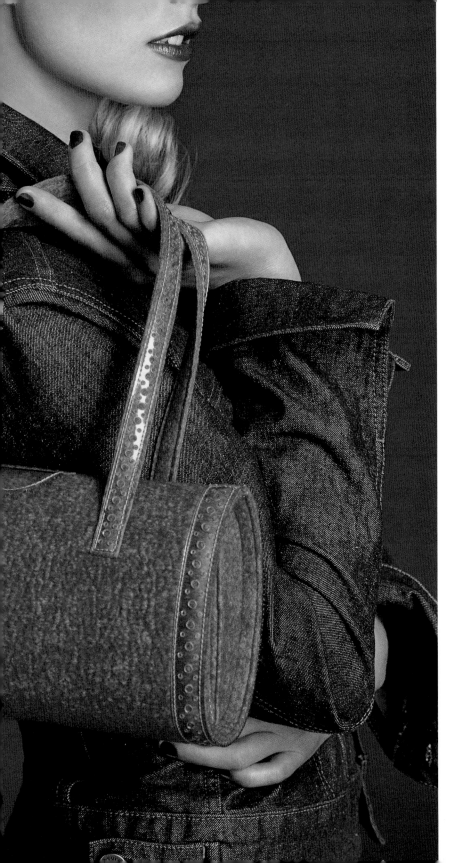

BREAK THE LATENESS HABIT.
ARRIVING MORE THAN THIRTY
MINUTES LATE TO A PARTY IS
NOT FASHIONABLE.

TO MAKE ROOM FOR THE NEW,
**THROW AWAY THE TWO PAIRS
OF SHOES** YOU HARDLY WORE
LAST WINTER.

23

**AVOID THE USE OF
PROFESSIONAL JARGON IN
CASUAL CONVERSATIONS.**
SAYING IT ALL WITH SIMPLE
WORDS—THAT'S STYLE.

25 **RESOLE YOUR FAVORITE PAIR OF BOOTS** BEFORE THE BAD WEATHER SETS IN.

26 GET A PAIR OF PROFESSIONAL TWEEZERS.

27 **BUY A NEW SWEATER** IN ONE OF THE COLORS OF THE SEASON: BRONZE, RUST, TOBACCO, CHOCOLATE, CAPPUCCINO.

ADDING THE STYLISH EXTRAS

Once you've established a foundation of simple, well-made, modern clothes, then stock up on accessories to express your own personal style—whether it be whimsical, trendy, ethnic, minimalist, or classic. Accessories are often less expensive than clothes, and they stay in style longer.

SHOES AND ACCESSORIES Both are critical to your overall appearance. They are even more important than clothing. Stylish accessories in elegant materials and modern designs can make a plain outfit work.

* **SHOES ARE THE FINISHING TOUCH,** the last thing you put on. Dress first before deciding what to wear on your feet. The shape of your shoes must complement your entire silhouette.
* **SHOES SHOULD EMBRACE THE FOOT.** The curve of the foot must be respected: Square toes are less elegant, because the foot is pointed.
* **SHOES SHOULD NEVER LOOK HEAVY,** though boots, worn with skirts, can be very elegant.
* **KEEP YOUR SHOES SHINED—ALWAYS.**
* **YOUR ACCESSORIES SHOULD FEEL WEIGHTLESS.** They should not weigh you down in any shape or form.
* **NEVER WEAR AN OUTRAGEOUS HAT,** unless it complements your face.
* **DO NOT WEAR TOO MUCH GOLD.** A no-no: wearing gold jewelry at the same time as sunglasses with gold-tone decorations.
* **DON'T EVEN ENTERTAIN THE THOUGHT** of allowing your glasses to dangle at the end of a chain around your neck.

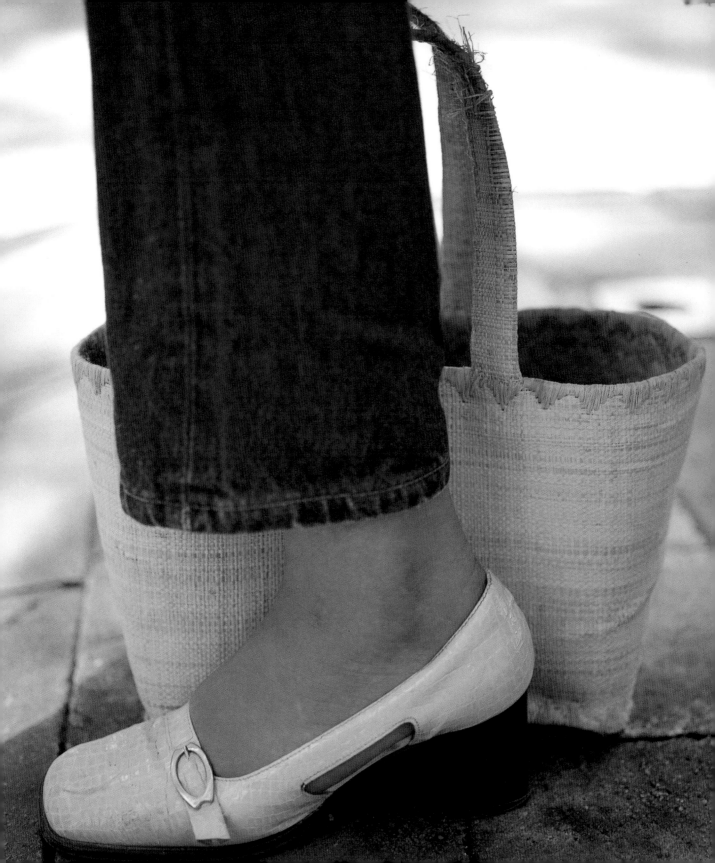

GREAT CUTS FOR CHILDREN

In September, I see more of my clients' families and significant others than any other month. Their children are going back to school, and their husbands and boyfriends are buckling down to work, just as they are. Everybody needs a bit of an overhaul. As with women's hair, the simplest routine is always the best, and the shape of the cut is everything. Children spend a great deal less time on their hair than women do, so a cut with real style is doubly important.

I've cut the hair of children of nearly every age, and my rule of thumb is, don't take them to a salon until they're at least five. It's just too unpleasant for all involved. There are special kids' salons that offer all kinds of enter-

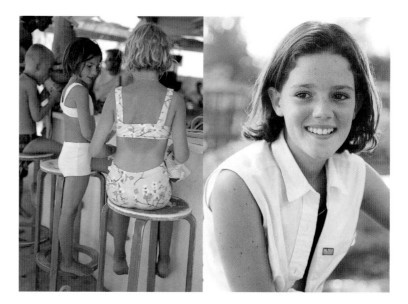

JUST LIKE ADULTS, CHILDREN NEED TO UPDATE
THEIR HAIRSTYLES FOR THE NEW SCHOOL YEAR.

page 216

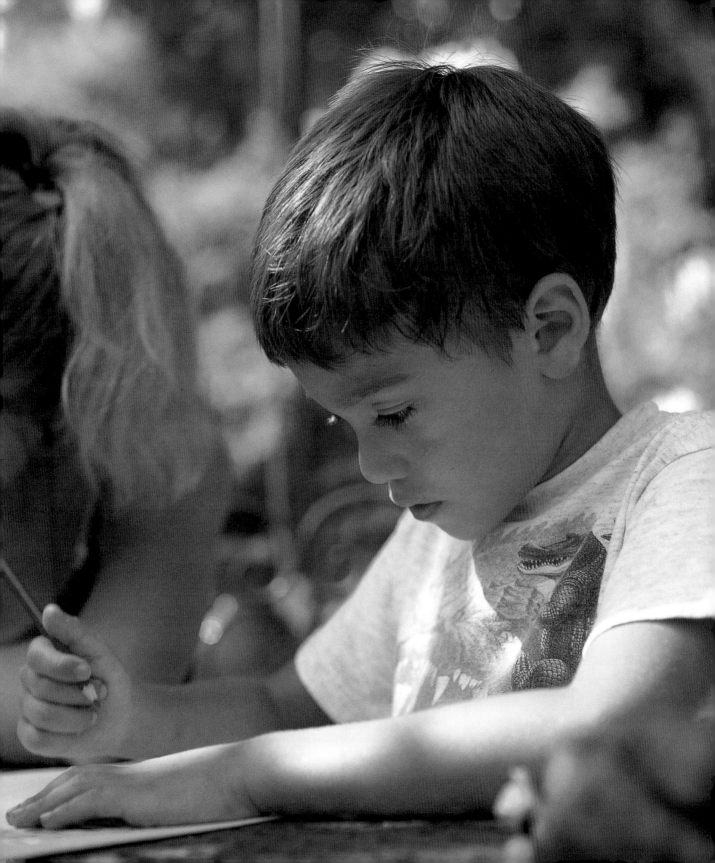

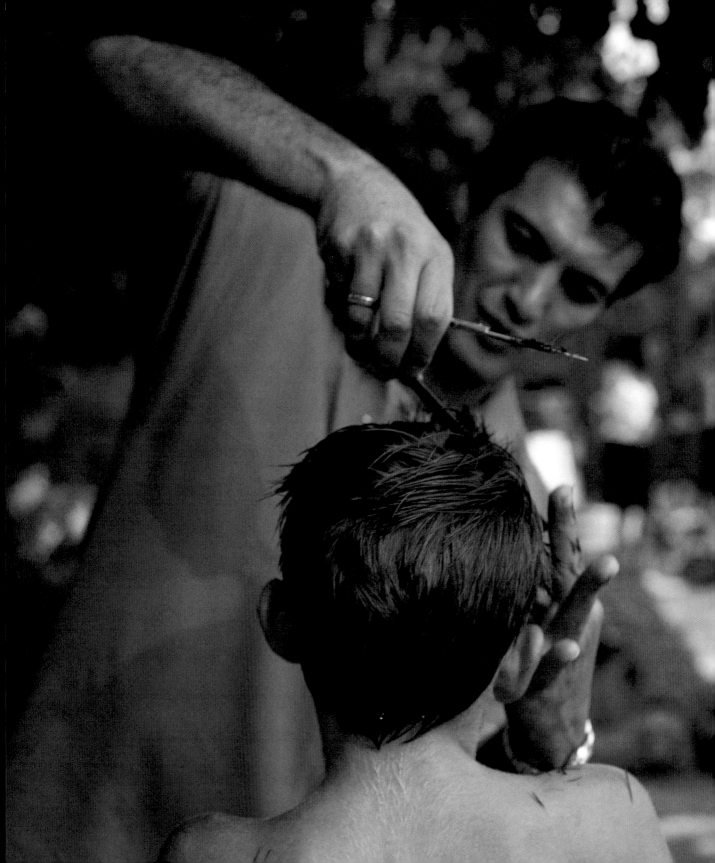

tainment, and even then, before four or five, it can be a disaster. Kids just don't have the attention span to sit still for a real cut. Above all, you want the experience to be a good one.

I remember getting haircuts growing up: I hated them. I'd go to the barber and he'd use these sharp, scary-looking razors, and my neck would itch. Whether you're in a salon or doing it yourself, make sure the child's hair is completely wet. Dry hair itches.

* Bobs are wonderful for little girls, whether their hair is straight or curly, because they are versatile. You can let them swing free, or pull them back with small barrettes or hairbands.
* Children are cute with hair parted in the middle, or hair cut square, because their faces are soft, regular, and symmetrical.
* Boys need cuts with a little more character than do girls. Boys' hair shouldn't be so short they look like they're in the Marines. Let them enjoy their hair.
* Trendy haircuts, like long tails at the back of a boy's head, look ridiculous on children (as they usually do on adults, as well).

TRY TO MAKE THE HAIR-CUTTING EXPERIENCE
FUN FOR YOUR CHILD BY VARYING THE PLACE
OR TIME—OUTDOORS IS PERFECT!

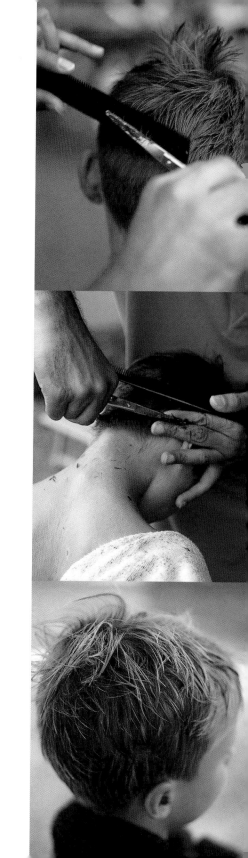

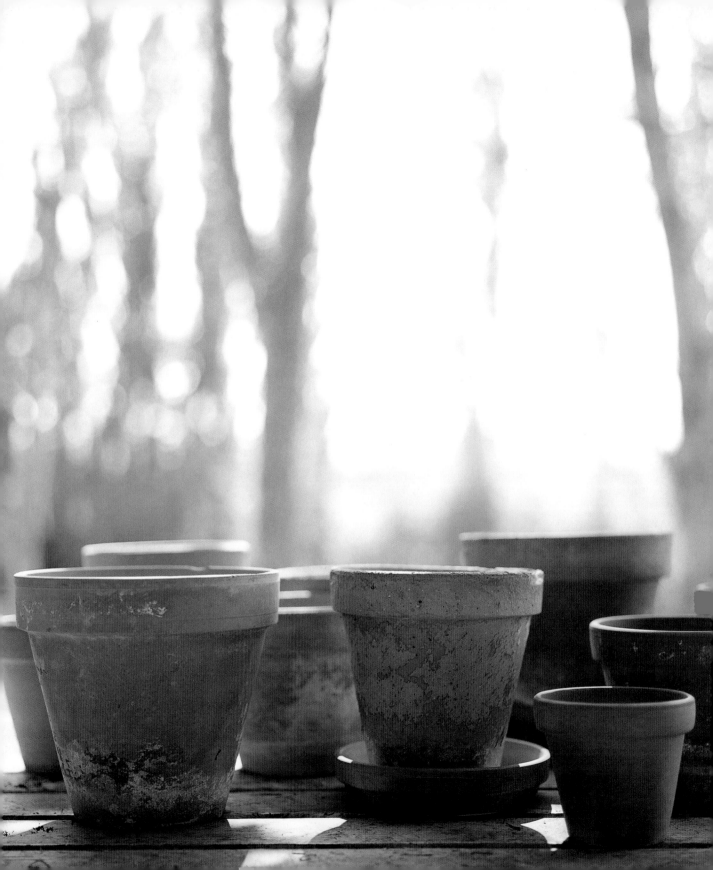

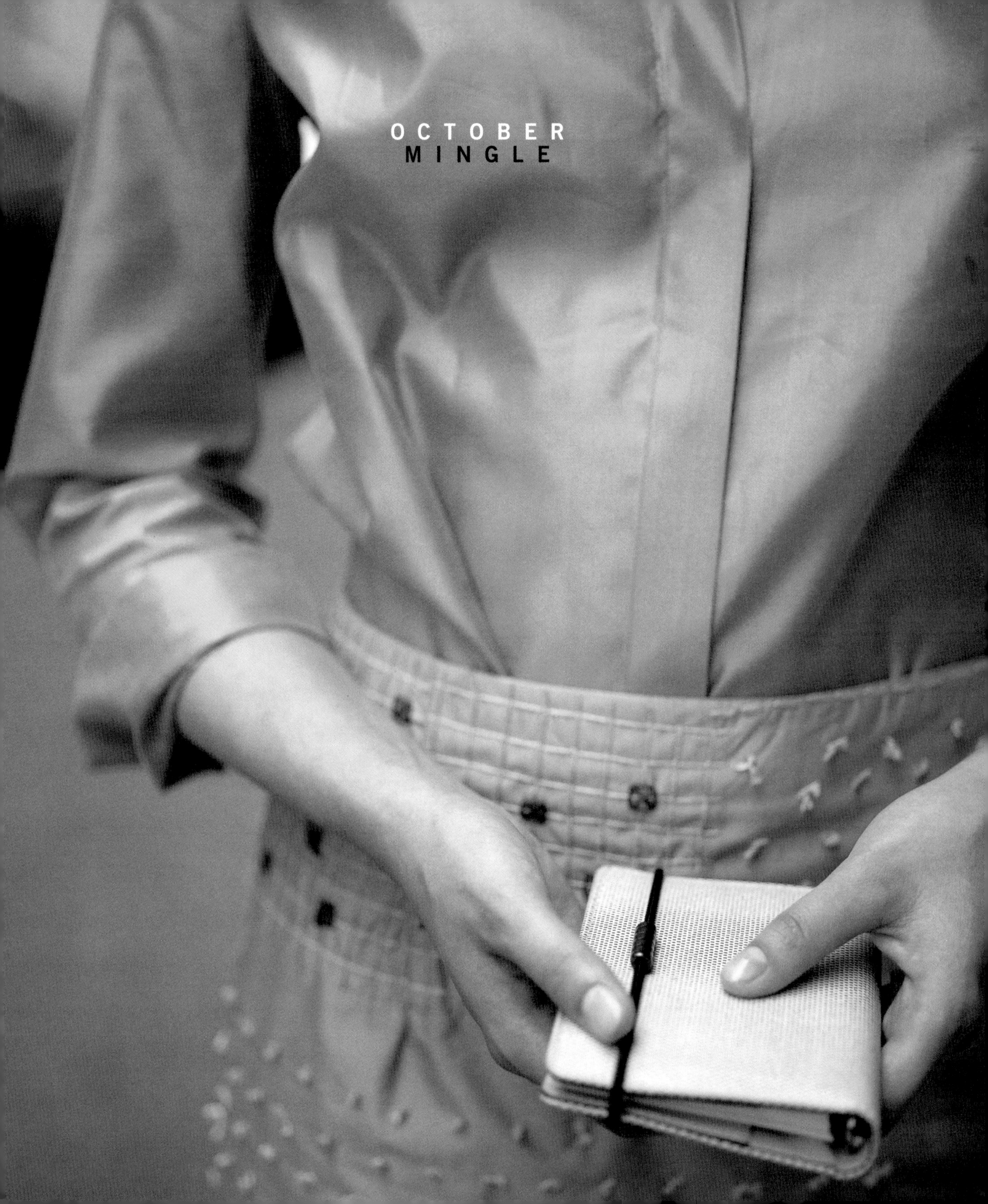

OCTOBER
MINGLE

ORGANIZE YOUR CLOSET BY COMPLEMENTARY TEXTURES: CORDUROY WITH FLANNEL, TWILL WITH LINEN, AND CASHMERE WITH WOOL.

1

BUY A NEW WHITE COTTON SHIRT OR TWO TO WEAR UNDER YOUR SUIT JACKETS.

2

HAVE A MAKEUP LESSON IN A SALON. GET ACQUAINTED WITH SOME OF THE NEWEST BEAUTY PRODUCTS. NEW TEXTURES ARE SOMETIMES MORE INTERESTING THAN NEW COLORS.

3

Though we all complain about it, we love to be too busy. Time flies when you hardly have time to think. Just yesterday, for instance, you looked at your calendar and realized that it was already October. What happened to September? Before you know it, Thanksgiving will be here! You shudder at the thought of all the social engagements, dinner parties, let's-get-together-for-lunch promises, and invitations you can't refuse. This is madness, yet you wouldn't want to miss any of it.

In order to enjoy the excitement of the season, you must learn to unwind as you go. You can't be expected to remain sane if you don't give yourself room to stretch and breathe. In New York, I go to the Boat Basin in Central Park first thing in the morning, even before breakfast. Somehow, gazing at the placid surface of the water gives me a healthy perspective on my day.

RIGHT: BEFORE LEAVING HOME FOR A BIG EVENING, TAKE A FEW MOMENTS TO RELAX WITH SOMEONE YOU LOVE.

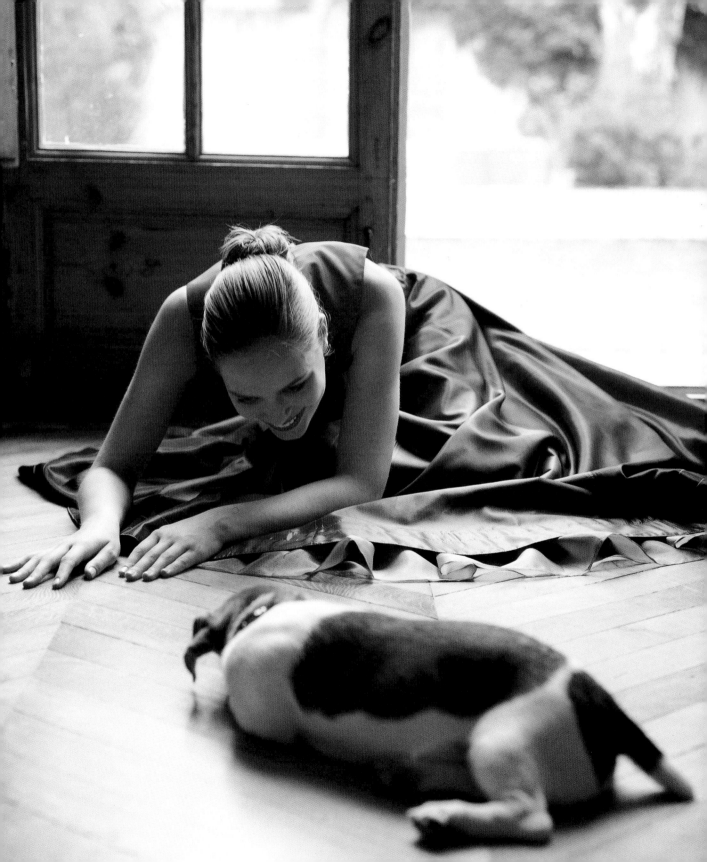

ADAPT. PEOPLE WHO ARE FLEXIBLE HAVE MORE STYLE THAN PEOPLE WHO TRY TO CONTROL EVERYTHING.

4

Asking your mother-in-law to respect your privacy is fine—as long as the request is delivered by your husband.

—JUDITH MARTIN
(MISS MANNERS)

5

REMEMBER A NEW JOKE TO TELL FRIENDS AND RELATIVES. IT RELAXES EVERYONE.

6

Occasionally, one needs to lose the notion of time. Better to be late and feel great than to be punctual and in a bad mood. If you see that you are running behind, call to apologize and, if need be, to reschedule your appointment. It's not the end of the world. Given a chance, most of us are glad for a reprieve and can use an extra hour to catch up. Remember this when others are late—don't begrudge them.

One of the delusions of modern life is thinking that you can escape it all in a vacation home. I used to have a house on the beach, but eventually I gave it up in order to regain my sanity. The routine of going there every weekend was stressful: There were simply too many organizational problems. Having friends come to visit created a lot of work. I found myself using precious leisure time to go grocery shopping for a houseful of people. I love to cook—I even like doing the dishes—but the responsibility of doing it all the time and for a crowd is too much for anyone who has a career and a family.

There is only one solution: Learn to deal with the pressure of a full work and social life by taking short breaks now and then. Make time for unexpected invitations, multiple engagements, conflicting schedules, and for your own private dawdling impulses.

Here are my suggestions for making the most of your social life:

* **Once a day, give priority to what you feel you need.**
* **Don't create problems if you can help it.**
* **Remember that people who are rude are in fact insecure.**
* **Take the time to talk with children.**
* **Don't wait to be asked. Give freely.**
* **Don't finish other people's sentences.**
* **Be nice, but every so often speak up for what you believe.**
* **Don't turn everything into a project.**
* **Make it a ritual to stop regularly for tea or coffee at your favorite neighborhood bistro.**

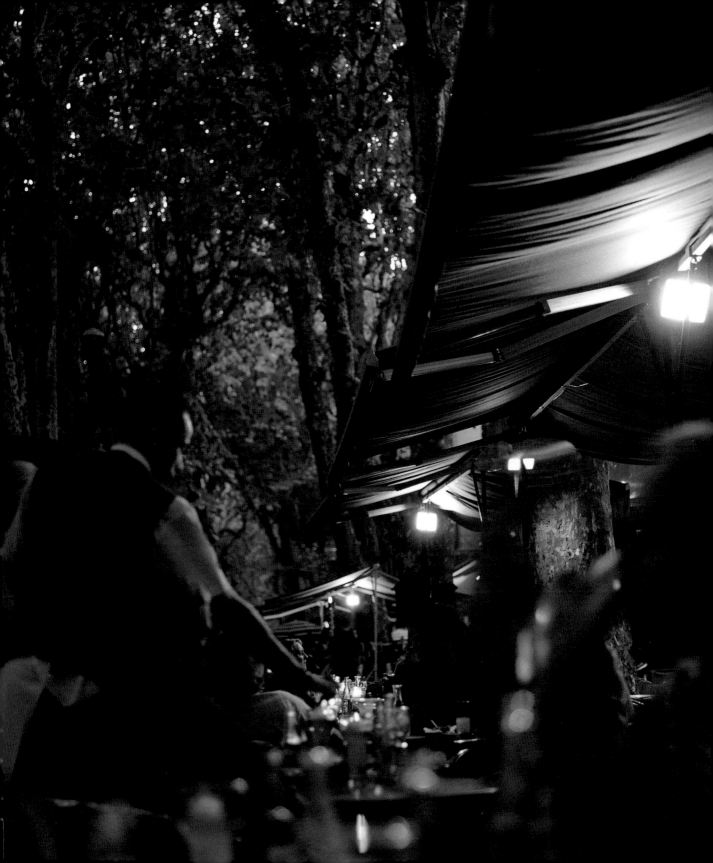

7

TO EASE THE THROBBING OF A HEADACHE, RUB HALF A LIME OVER YOUR FOREHEAD.

8

Baby a man when he is sick or has a hangover, but leave him alone when he is in a bad mood.

—MAE WEST

9

EXPERIMENT WITH A NEW RICH-BROWN EYE SHADOW, EXTENDING IT TOWARD YOUR TEMPLES TO ELONGATE THE SHAPE OF YOUR EYES.

ELEGANT GLAMOUR FOR
BIG NIGHTS

October is the beginning of a more formal social season. The whole idea of getting all dressed up is fresh and thrilling. Most of us look forward to a party with an attitude of enchantment and self-indulgence. But having fun doesn't necessarily mean going over the top. Even in the dead of winter, dressing up should involve the same sense of simplicity and ease that a casual summer afternoon might inspire. Live by that rule and you'll never end up overdone, overdressed, or uncomfortable.

Like everyone else, I cherish the memory of my parents going out at night. I always think about them when I'm getting ready for a big event. For a child, watching Mom and Dad transform into glamorous creatures is a formative experience. I was lucky: Every year in Aix there was, and still is, a two-week-long Opera Festival, jam-packed with black-tie events. The displays of incredible style there forever colored my view of formal dressing. You'd see some of the most amazing gowns, everything from fluffy bouffant confections to fitted long dresses. One woman would show up in a deep, dahlia-red, strapless gown, fitted to the waist, with swirls of fabric falling to the floor. She'd have little beaded heels, and a necklace of tiny diamonds and red sapphires. Standing next to her would be another, equally stylish woman in a midnight-blue fitted dress, beaded all over and cut at the knee, maybe with a pair of ballet flats and a diamond solitaire.

RIGHT: GILLIAN ANDERSON HAS AN UNDERSTATED STYLE THAT I ADMIRE. WITH HER FANTASTIC RED HAIR, SHE LOVES COLOR AND COLOR LOVES HER. FOR THE 1999 SAG AWARDS, I CREATED SOME CURLS IN HER HAIR, TWISTING THEM TO THE TOP OF HER HEAD AND LETTING SOME HANG DOWN IN BACK.

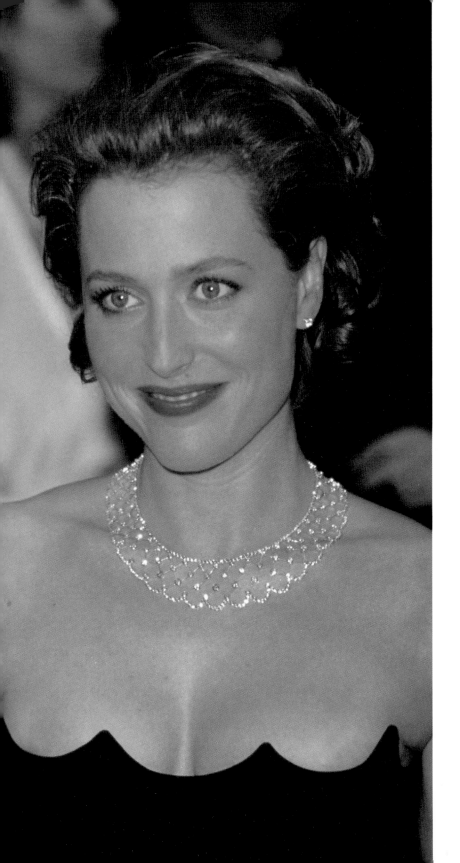

EVENING ELEGANCE

A strong sense of simplicity, coupled with the knowledge that a black-tie event should be a very special night—and therefore merit a little extra effort—is the route to true evening elegance. The rest is easy. Here are the must-have elements:

* HAIR OFF THE FACE, but not too severe

* A VERY BEAUTIFUL DRESS

* COLOR, if not in your dress then your accessories

* VERY PRETTY SHOES, preferably strappy heels

* A LITTLE TOUCH of jewelry

* AN ELEGANT SHAWL

* A SMALL EVENING BAG

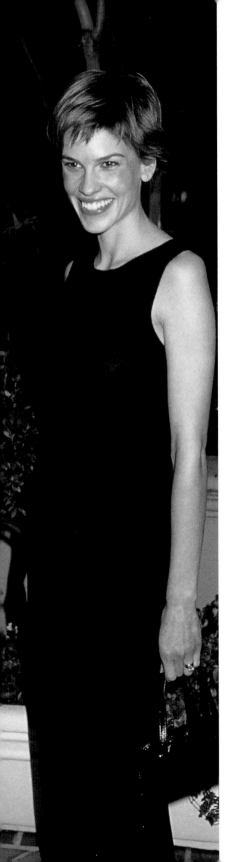

My mother managed to look just as sensational, but with a simpler attire. She'd brush her long hair into a ponytail, twist it up and around into a chignon, and secure it with a few hairpins. Then she'd put on a little eyeliner and mascara, brush on some lipstick, dab a bit of it on the apple of each cheek, smudging it lightly, and that was it. She'd put together something like a sleeveless top in ivory silk, with black, shaped trousers and a great belt, all wrapped up with a cashmere shawl. Just before the shawl, she'd touch her wrists and neck with her perfume—which I love to this day—L'heure Bleue, by Guerlain.

GETTING IN THE MOOD

Too often going to a party, which is supposed to be fun, turns into a last-minute nightmare as you struggle to get ready. When a man and a woman have to get dressed at the same time, especially if they are sharing a mirror, there is even more tension. Since the act of dressing up for an event sets the tone for the rest of the evening, try to make it a pleasure. You don't get to do this every day—revel in the experience.

A man and a woman should not dress together in the same room. I always try to be ready before the woman I'm escorting, so I can bring her a drink, change the music, help her with whatever she might need. I consider that my role is to facilitate her preparation. I leave her alone. I do not offer to help, but I am available. A women can be easily flustered when she gets dressed, and a man should be careful not to make her feel even more nervous by getting in her way.

LEFT: HILARY SWANK KNOWS HOW TO RELAX AND PREPARE FOR A GALA EVENT. PRIOR TO THE 2000 ACADEMY AWARDS, WHERE SHE WAS HONORED WITH A MUCH-DESERVED OSCAR, SHE VISITED MY SALON IN BEVERLY HILLS FOR A DAY OF BEAUTY.

* **HAVE A REFRESHING DRINK:** an iced tea, sparkling water, or a glass of champagne (if you are not the one driving).
* **EAT A LITTLE SOMETHING AS WELL,** preferably finger food that is easy to eat with a toothpick and doesn't get your hands dirty. I suggest something with a bit of protein, like a few slices of grilled chicken, cubes of cooked fish, some fruit with goat cheese, even a quick scrambled egg. Your energy will hold up better over a long evening, and you won't go overboard on the hors d'oeuvres.
* **DON'T TURN ON THE TV AS YOU DRESS.** Instead, play great music. Classic jazz will put you in the mood, and so will chamber music.
* **UNPLUG THE PHONE** (unless you have kids, of course; a parent is always a parent, even in a tuxedo). The reason most of us are late is usually because of last-minute phone calls.
* **MAKE SURE THERE IS A CHAIR IN YOUR DRESSING ROOM** and sit down while putting on your clothes or adjusting your hair or your makeup.
* **YOU NEED AMPLE LIGHT** as you are putting your makeup on, but be sure to check how it will look in the dimmer light typical of most parties. You may decide you need a touch more color.
* **USE SCENTED OIL OR BODY LOTION:** It will make your skin wonderful to touch. Then spray or splash your favorite eau de toilette or perfume. Use restraint—don't drown yourself in it.
* **DON'T LOOK AT THE RESULT UNTIL YOU'RE COMPLETELY DONE.** Finishing touches like mascara and accessories make all the difference. Evaluating your look too early can be disconcerting.

REPLACE STRAGGLY HOUSEPLANTS WITH NEW LUSH ONES.

10

AVOID GETTING STIFF HANDS FROM REPETITIVE TASKS BY OPENING AND CLOSING THEM UNDER WATER EACH TIME YOU WASH THEM.

11

TAKE ADVANTAGE OF THE INDIAN SUMMER TO HAVE ONE LAST PICNIC WITH FRIENDS. ON THE MENU: GRILLED VEGETABLES, POACHED SALMON, TARTE TATIN—AND A BOTTLE OF SAUVIGNON BLANC.

12

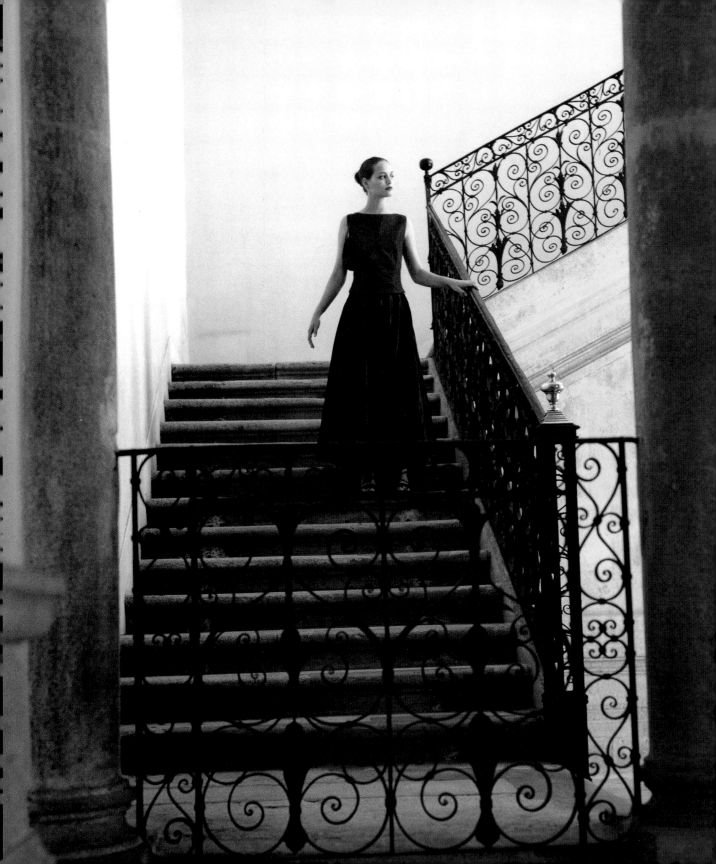

WHAT TO WEAR AND HOW TO WEAR IT

The best evening clothes are simply designed but made of luxurious materials. Elaborately pieced-together ensembles never work. Above all, you want to be comfortable, you want to be you.

Black is slimming and elegant, but because everyone wears it, it's hard to stand out in black. If you do choose black, give extra thought to your accessories. Wild patterns and prominent logos invariably flatter themselves more than they flatter you.

I believe that accessories define personal style even more than clothing does. Great shoes, as always, can turn a perfectly acceptable look into something sublime. But balance style with comfort: If you plan to be dancing for five hours, stilettos are hard to pull off. On the other hand, if most of the evening consists of a sit-down dinner, this might be your chance to wear something sexy and gorgeous and completely impractical.

Materials for shoes should reflect the spirit of the evening: Silk, velvet, *peau de soie,* satin, crystals . . . indulge your senses. Intricately embroidered flats say "evening" in a way that leather pumps never will.

Your jewelry, like your clothes, is a little flourish of style that should, above all, keep the focus on you. For this reason, I don't like statement jewelry: I want to remember the woman, not her ruby-and-sapphire-encrusted wedding-cake brooch. Similarly, beware of big earrings, chunky jewelry, necklaces like armor plates. Absolutely beautiful as sculpture, some pieces of jewelry should never be worn by human beings.

A good way to tell if the jewelry is right for you: Make sure it follows the contours of your neck or your wrist and accentuates their gracious curves. You'll never go wrong if you choose a simple necklace (even a classic pearl one), a little diamond, a hair stick, barrettes with pearls, or something small and precious in a great color that complements what you're wearing.

RESOLVE TO BUILD YOUR SELF-ESTEEM. DON'T PUT YOURSELF DOWN, EVEN IN JEST.

13

Dreams are necessary to live.
—ANAÏS NIN

14

INDULGE IN A HYDRO-THERAPY BODY POLISH. IT'S AN INVIGORATING SHOWER MASSAGE THAT EXFOLIATES YOUR SKIN TO RESTORE ITS NATURAL GLOW.

15

16 SET ASIDE TIME TO SORT OUT YOUR SUMMER SNAP-SHOTS. MAKE A SCRAPBOOK INSTEAD OF THROWING THEM INTO A SHOE BOX. INCLUDE HANDWRITTEN NOTES, SCRAPS OF FABRIC, MATCHBOOK COVERS, AND PRESSED FLOWERS.

17 WHEN APPLYING MASCARA, ROTATE YOUR BRUSH TO SEPARATE AND LENGTHEN YOUR LASHES AT THE SAME TIME.

18 USE FRENCH WORDS IN CONVERSATION SPARINGLY, EVEN IF YOU SPEAK IT FLUENTLY. SHOWING OFF IS ANNOYING.

Day watches don't work for evening. Period. End of conversation. If you don't have an evening watch, simply go without (you can carry your daytime watch in your bag). For an evening watch, the strap should be thinner and flatter than the one on your day watch. The face should be smaller, more jewel-like.

Evening bags should be gorgeous, elegant, and refined, but they don't need to be as serious as a bag for everyday life. They should reflect the mood of your outfit, or have a great sense of fun. Your evening bag should be soft, made of rich fabric; harder materials like metal or even everyday leather just don't look right. Whimsical details and bright colors on an evening bag can make an otherwise boring outfit into something fabulous.

WHAT TO TAKE

Don't pack too much in an evening bag. That feeling of carrying almost nothing, leaving all your usual burdens at home, is more intoxicating than the finest champagne. You instantly feel lighter, more spirited. Here is all a lady needs in her evening purse:

✳ ONE CREDIT CARD

✳ ONE LIPSTICK (or crayon, or gloss)

✳ A TINY COMPACT with mirror

✳ READING GLASSES, if appropriate

✳ MINTS

✳ MAD MONEY. Be sure to have small bills for bathroom attendants, valets, etc.

✳ A MINIATURE CAMERA if you like, to record special moments

✳ NO CELL PHONE, PLEASE! (unless you're a parent, of course)

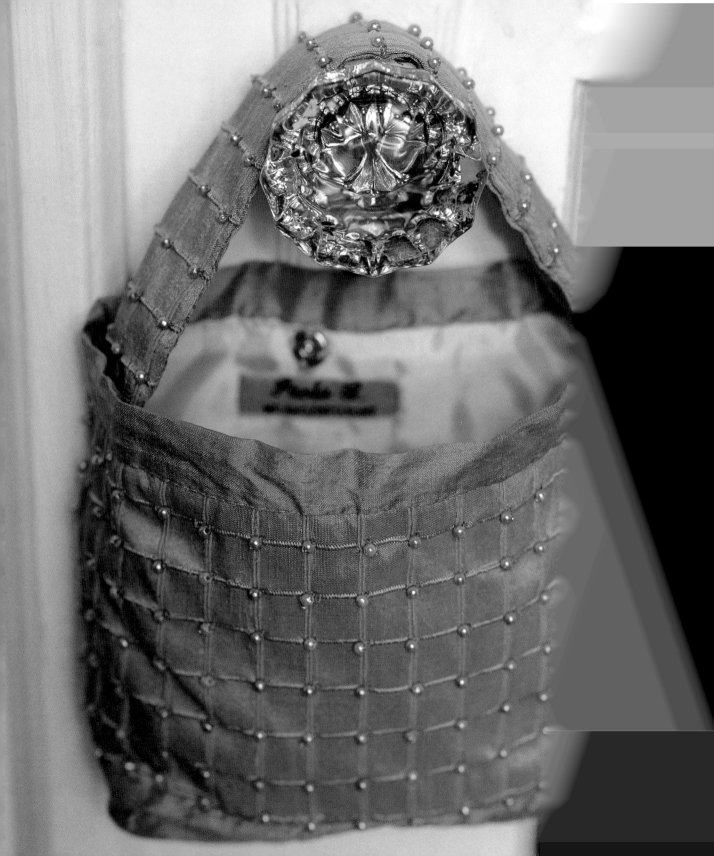

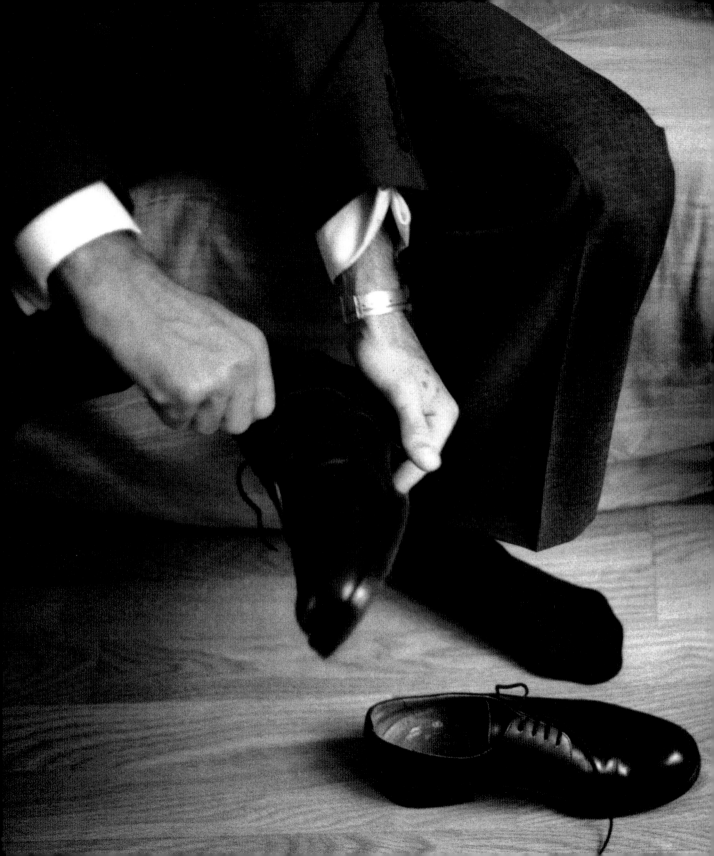

FORMAL ATTIRE FOR MEN

Women almost always influence their escorts' style in some way. Your advice is generally going to be heeded, so make yourself perfectly clear:

* **TUXEDOS SHOULD BE WORN WITH A WHITE SHIRT.** Black shirts make even the most handsome man look like a two-bit gangster.
* **FOR TRADITIONAL EVENTS** like most charity events in New York, I wear a double-breasted tuxedo with a bow tie. In L.A., where styles are less conservative and slightly less formal, a three-button tuxedo with a long pewter tie is my uniform.
* **THE TIE SHOULD NEVER** show anywhere around the neck except where it falls from the collar opening.
* **HAVE FUN WITH CUFFLINKS.** Some of the most elegant have a bit of wit, but the suggestion of a more daring color in a cufflink with semi-precious or precious stones can be extremely stylish. Large cufflinks, however amusing they might be, are no good.
* **MEN SHOULD CHANGE THEIR WATCHES** when they're going out: A softer, flatter face, perhaps something in gold or silver with a mother-of-pearl face. The idea, for everyone, is a little evening style.

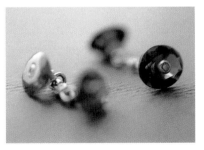

ABOVE: ONE OF MY FAVORITE PAIRS OF CUFFLINKS.
LEFT: SHOES MAKE THE MAN.
MAKE SURE THEY ARE ALWAYS WELL SHINED.

Dare to be naïve.
—BUCKMINSTER FULLER

19

ARE YOUR NAILS BREAKING?
YOUR BODY MAY BE TELLING
YOU THAT YOU NEED MORE
ZINC, CALCIUM, POTASSIUM,
AND VITAMIN C.

20

A COUPLE OF TIMES DURING
THE DAY, **GET UP FROM YOUR
DESK,** STRETCH, MASSAGE
YOUR NECK, YAWN.

21

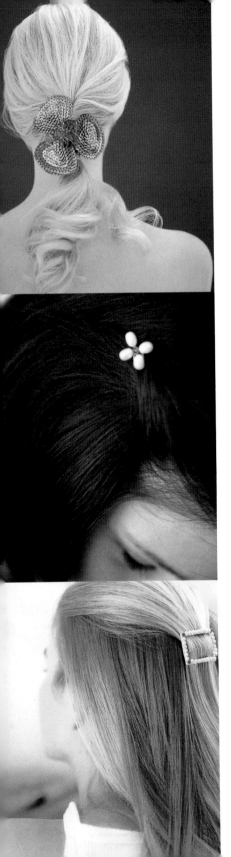

EVENING HAIR

You'll never be prettier than you are in the soft glowing light of a fancy party. Hide your face behind heavy locks or thick bangs, and you'll miss an opportunity to reveal the most elegant side of your personality.

To get your hair off your face, a little chignon secured with a barrette is the simplest, and often sexiest, of all updos. All you have to do is pull your hair into a ponytail, twist it, pull it up toward the top of your head, and secure it with a barrette. Once you get the knack of it, you won't even need a mirror to create this most sophisticated look.

Some women—I think of Gwyneth Paltrow, for instance, or Nicole Kidman —look spectacular with their hair down for evening. This is a look that's particularly hot with very simple, shoulder-baring clothes; the combination of bare shoulders and long, healthy-looking hair is all-out sexy. If you plan to wear your hair down, by all means, blow it dry, with special attention to get volume at the roots and shine on the ends (see May, "The Big Blowout"). Use a round brush to flip the ends just a bit, it leaves a more polished look that's perfect for evening.

Even the shortest hair should get a little extra attention in preparing for a big evening out. That "extra" could be something as simple as more shine (pomade or hair cream, applied a little bit at a time as you style, is the best way to achieve this), or it might involve accessories: a little ribbon, perhaps, or a bobby pin with a diamond on it. Pay particular attention to your earrings when you've got short hair: It's an opportunity for them to sparkle.

EVENING HAIR AND MAKEUP ARE ALL ABOUT ACCENTS—
HAIR ACCESSORIES AND COLOR.

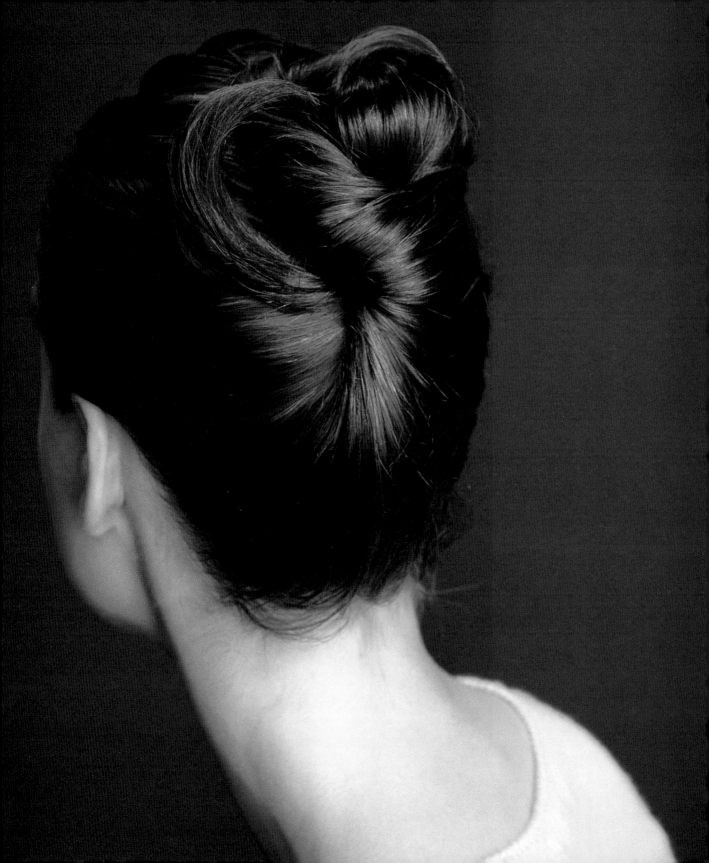

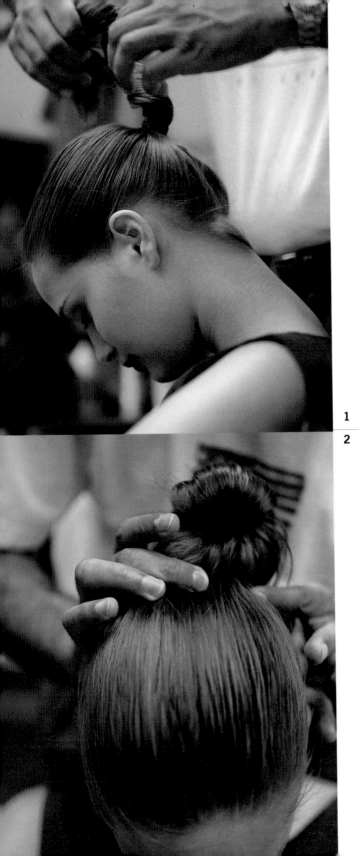
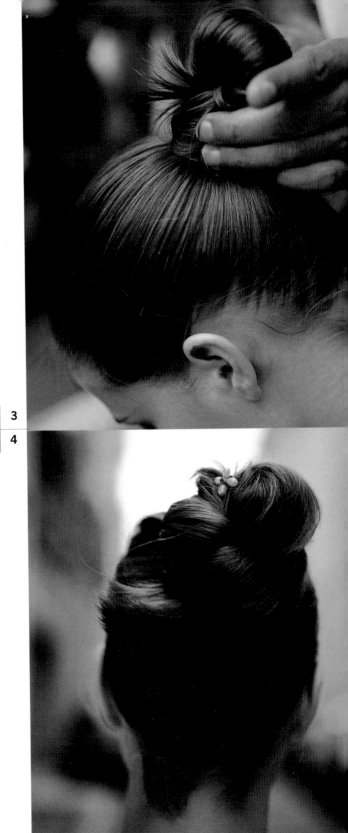

1 | 3
2 | 4

THE EVENING UPDO

A smooth updo, dressed with a subtle, small hair ornament, is an easy way to get a fast, festive look. It's just right for a fancy birthday party, gallery opening, premiere, or charity event. Once you have the knack of it, you won't even need a mirror to create this most sophisticated look:

∗ **BLOW-DRY YOUR HAIR** to bring out its shine and get rid of the frizz.

∗ **APPLY JUST A HINT OF POMADE** or gel to control unruly strands.

∗ **SLICK YOUR HAIR BACK** with both hands, put it in a low ponytail, and hold it firmly in place in your left hand.

∗ **TWIST THE GATHERED HAIR** into a loop around the index finger of your right hand.

∗ **PULL THE LOOP UP GENTLY** toward the top of your head.

∗ **SECURE THE BUN** with a barrette, a jeweled comb, or with a couple of big hairpins.

∗ **AS LONG AS THE MASS OF YOUR HAIR** feels secured, allow a couple of loose strands to escape from the bun. If need be, slick them with a little bit of pomade to give them more definition.

BUY BEAUTIFUL BOOKS, EVEN IF YOU DON'T HAVE TIME TO READ THEM ALL. THEY WILL MAKE YOUR HOME FEEL COMFORTABLE. ROOMS WITHOUT BOOKS ARE AS IMPERSONAL AS HOTEL ROOMS.

22

PICK AN OUTFIT IN A MAGAZINE BEFORE YOU PICK IT FROM THE RACK. HAVE AN IMAGE IN YOUR MIND OF WHAT YOU ARE LOOKING FOR BEFORE YOU EMBARK ON YOUR NEXT SHOPPING SPREE.

23

INDULGE IN A BOX OF HARD-MILLED BODY SOAPS.

24

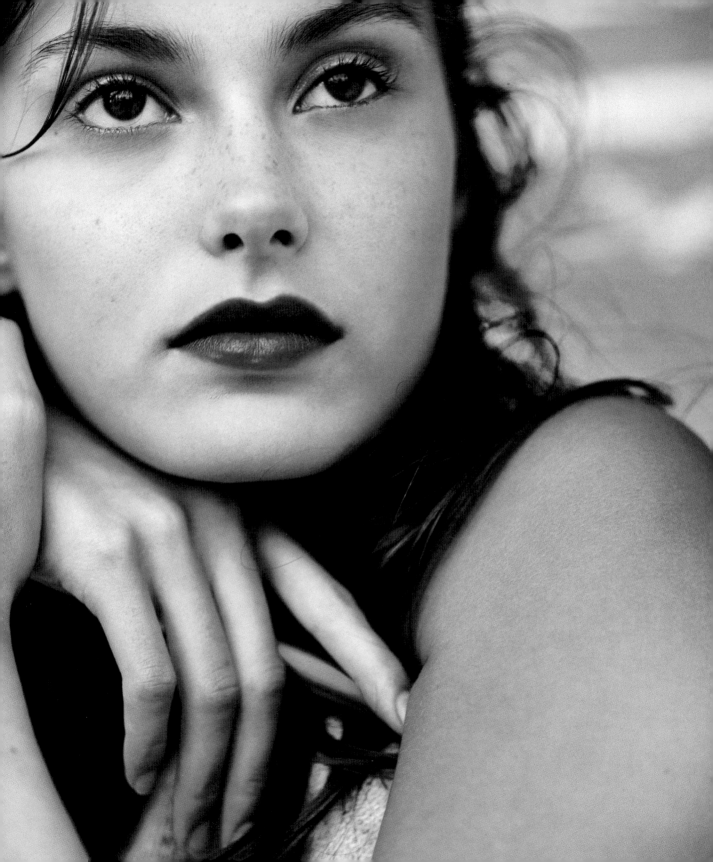

EVENING MAKEUP

Even if you barely wear makeup during the day, putting a little more on makes you look and feel more glamorous. Remember that lights at evening events are generally low, so you'll need a touch more makeup if you want it to show up. The other thing to remember when you're going for drama is to keep it simple. A full face of makeup really isn't modern, nor is it sexy. My approach is to focus on one aspect of your face, with a great shade of lipstick, perhaps, or really dramatic, smoky eyes, but never both. However, it's important to balance the color on your face. If you pair extreme eyes with completely bare lips, it will look like you forgot something. Remember the following:

* **PERFECTING YOUR SKIN WITH CONCEALER,** foundation, and powder is always a good idea. Refer back to the tips on pages 200–201.

* **SOME WOMEN LOVE A DEWY, VERY NATURAL SKIN AT NIGHT,** and they reason that by the time it fades, who cares? If you're this type of person, use light but creamy foundation formulas, and very little powder. Shimmer sticks or powders (subtle ones) can also enhance the dewy look.

* **OTHER WOMEN LIKE THEIR MAKEUP TO STAY ON** for the entire evening. There are many long-lasting products on the market, but none are more crucial than powder. A supermodel known for her always-perfect-looking skin told me this: Once you've done your makeup, smooth a powder puff across a pan of pressed powder, then press it firmly into your skin. A minute later, dip a brush in loose powder, blow off the excess, and dust your face with it. The effect will be as natural as ever, but your makeup will simply not come off.

* **DON'T WEAR LIPSTICK THAT HAS TO BE TOUCHED UP CONSTANTLY.** You want to be thinking about all the fun you're having, not your lipstick.

IF YOUR SHOULDER BAG HANGS PAST YOUR HIP, HAVE A SHOEMAKER SHORTEN THE STRAP.

25

INSTEAD OF FLOWERS, **COLLECT SOME GREAT FALLEN LEAVES,** AND PRESS THEM IN A DICTIONARY.

26

KEEP UP THE HIGHLIGHTS YOU GOT NATURALLY THIS SUMMER WITH PROFESSIONAL HELP.

27

28 SEND A PACKAGE OF SMALL LUXURIES TO FRIENDS WHO LIVE FAR AWAY. WITH A LITTLE LUCK, THEY'LL GET IT IN TIME FOR CHRISTMAS.

29 KEEP SEVERAL BOTTLES OF GOOD CHAMPAGNE IN THE FRIDGE FOR IMPROMPTU HOLIDAY GET-TOGETHERS.

30 TAKE A LONG WALK WHILE THE WEATHER IS STILL MILD.

31 USE LIPBALM TO KEEP CUTICLES FROM BECOMING DRY OR CRACKED IN COLD WEATHER.

THE GALA FACE

A smoky eye and sexy lip can be perfect for parties. A dark eye, a little heavier than you would normally wear in the daytime, looks great in a candlelit setting. Don't go overboard with the shadow, as you could wind up looking like Cleopatra. And remember the secret to a smooth, dark eye is to blend, blend, blend. Here's one way to create stylish evening eyes.

＊ **EYES** Since much of the visual emphasis falls on the eyes, it's very important to have a clean brow. Groom your brow carefully and fill in your brow line with a pencil or powder shadow that matches your brow coloring. Use a deep, neutral eye pencil to line both the lid and under the eye. Gently smudge the line (without removing it entirely) to soften the look. Apply a shimmery neutral shadow over the entire lid and up to the brow bone. Choose a charcoal or rich brown shadow and, using a thin brush, apply the shadow on the top lid, keeping close to the lash line. The charcoal or brown shadow should sweep across the lid to the outer corner of the eye and just under the outer corner so that it forms a soft point. Blend well. Finish with two coats of black mascara, combing the lashes out between coats.

＊ **CHEEKS** Pick a pink, earthy tone and with a light hand apply the blush to the upper part of the apples of your cheeks. This will bring out the smoky eye and help bring the eyes and cheeks together.

＊ **LIPS** Choose a neutral red color for your lips to balance out the dark, smoky eye. A deep, rich brick red works well with most skin tones. After you have applied the color, finish with a touch of clear gloss in the center of the lower lip. This technique will make your mouth a little more plump and sexy.

＊ **NAILS** With a more made-up face, keep the nails very simple. A very subtle polish works well.

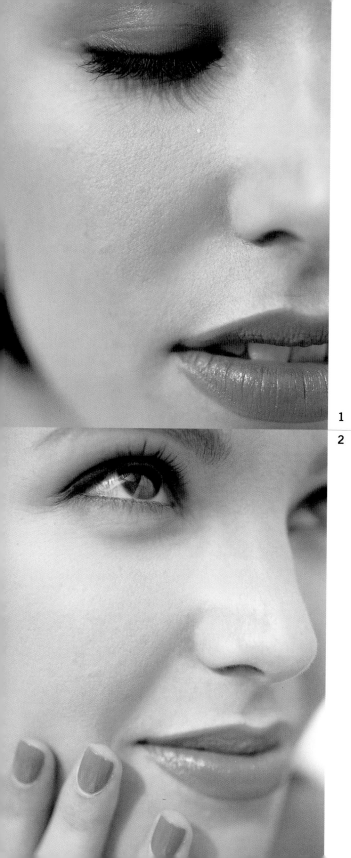

1
2
3

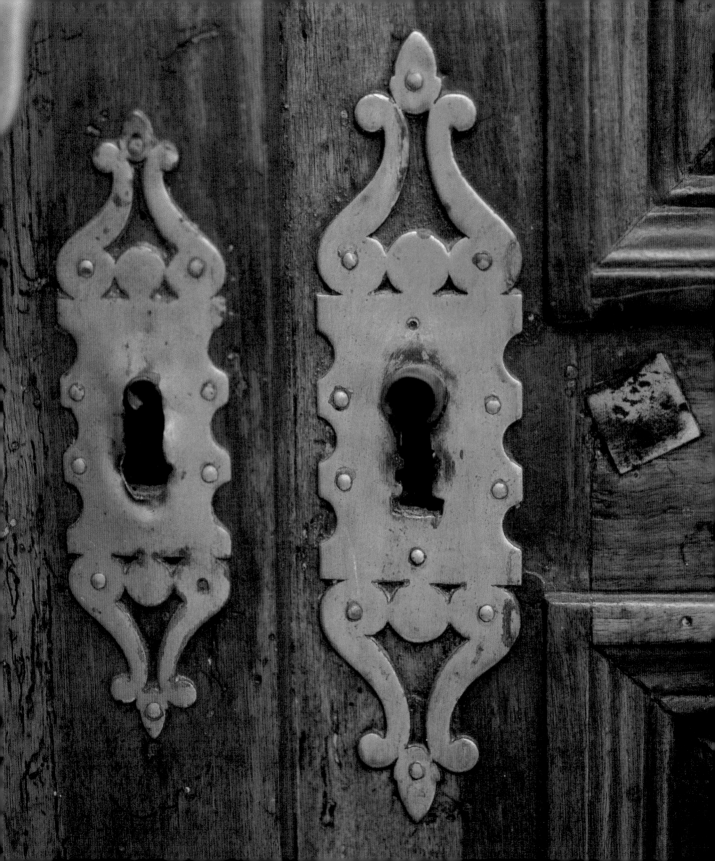

NOVEMBER
DE-STRESS

1 **BEGIN YOUR HOLIDAY SHOPPING NOW,** TO AVOID CROWDS AND STRESS.

2 **TREAT YOURSELF** TO A PRE-HOLIDAY AROMATIC DEEP CLEANSING FACIAL AT A NEW DAY SPA.

3 BUY A GREAT RED LIPSTICK FOR THE HOLIDAYS.

As months go, November sometimes loses its identity. With its promise of Christmas, Chanukah, and New Year's Eve, December beckons seductively; getting through the chilly, hectic, errand-filled days of November may seem like an exercise in problem solving. When will you get your Christmas shopping done? How can you ready your house for the flurry of guests and entertaining? What will you wear to the spate of parties you'll be attending? How can you keep yourself looking sleek and pretty and together when the days are crammed full?

In the last month or so, you've looked at so many fashion and beauty magazines, your head is spinning. Everywhere you turn, there is a new article telling you how to look better, dress better, feel better. By now you've learned so many new beauty "tricks" your morning hair-and-makeup routine takes twice as long as before—and still you're not entirely happy with

RIGHT: EVERYDAY TASKS CAN CONTRIBUTE TO FRAZZLED NERVES AS THE HOLIDAYS APPROACH.

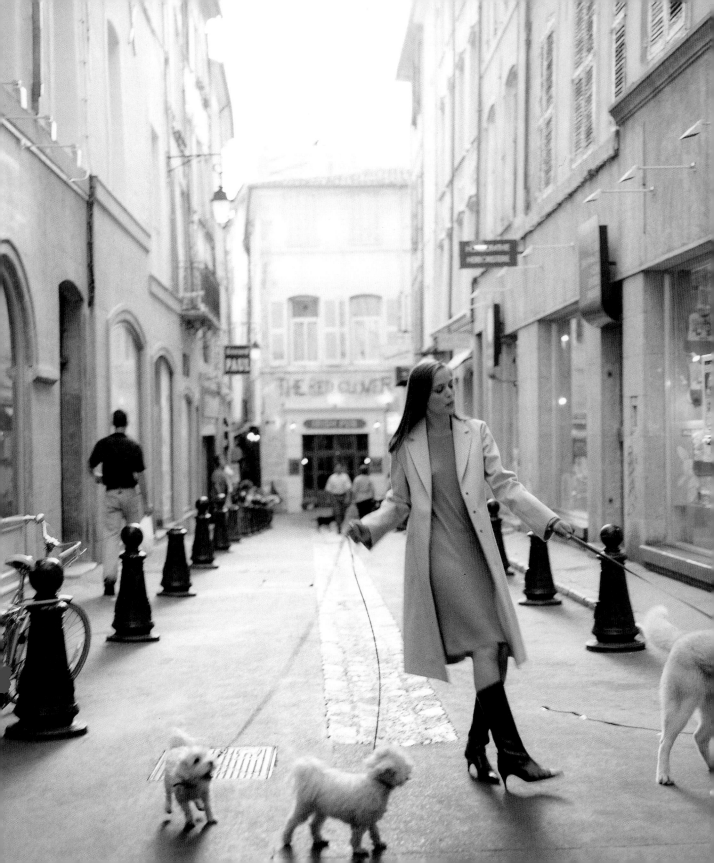

Wit is the only
wall / Between us
and the dark.

—MARK VAN DOREN

4

5 SLOW DOWN A LITTLE; YOU'LL
BE MORE EFFICIENT.

6 BUY A NEW AGENDA NOW;
YOU'LL BE MORE ORGANIZED
NEXT YEAR.

the results. You're way too busy for a major style overhaul, but everyone needs an arsenal of quick solutions for days when total indulgence is simply not possible. You need solutions—and fast.

But before you rush ahead to fix things up, take a moment for yourself. Exhale, relax your shoulders, straighten your spine, smile. If only you could see yourself now, you'd realize how attractive you are. Bringing out your own beauty is as simple as that.

LEARN TO LOOK AT YOURSELF IN MIRRORS

Too often we hate the frozen reflection we see in a mirror, and so we make rash decisions to correct flaws that don't even exist.

Don't just stare at yourself in the mirror in the morning. It's the least flattering moment of the day. To get an impression of how you look in real life, catch your reflection all through the day. You'll be pleasantly surprised.

When scrutinizing your image, run a hand through your hair. See how it feels. Notice what your hand does—it will naturally go to the problem spots:

* ARE YOU FLUFFING your hair or patting it down here and there? You can probably use a good trim.

* ARE YOU STROKING your jawline up and down and rubbing your cheekbones? You feel tired and should try to get a good night's sleep.

* ARE YOU STRAIGHTENING your posture? You need to exercise more often.

* LOOK INTO THE MIRROR before leaving your house to figure out what to eliminate—not what to add.

* REMOVE YOUR GOLD NECKLACE: It's too much flash for daytime.

* LOSE THE EXTRA TOTE BAG: Discipline yourself to carry less stuff. The lighter you travel, the better you look.

In fact, a mirror is something to glance at only occasionally, for small adjustments, just to check that indeed you look as good as you feel.

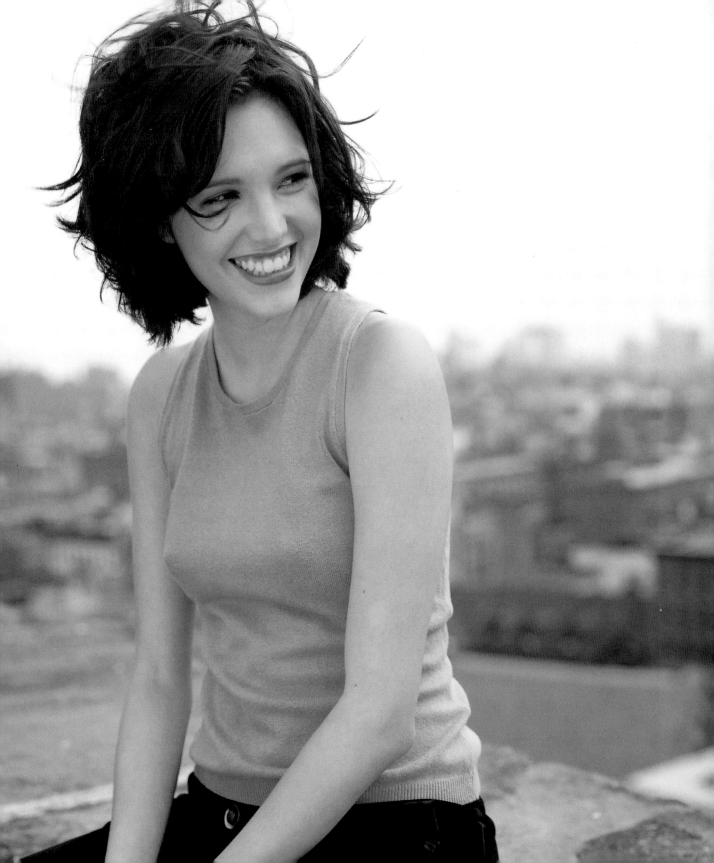

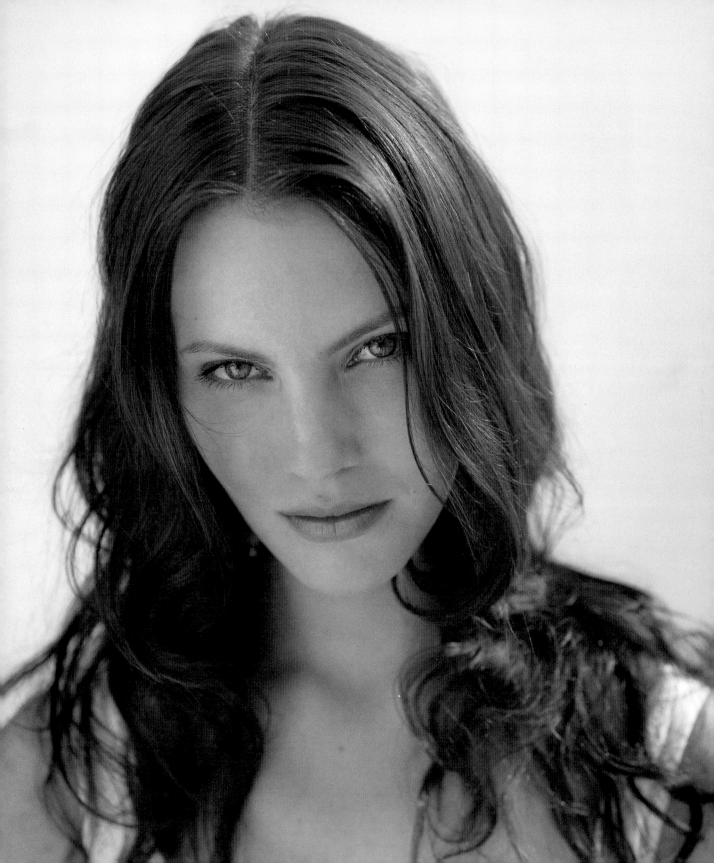

DEALING
WITH A BAD HAIR DAY

A bad hair day is usually, but not always, about unruly hair and frizz. When a bad hair day hits, the impulse is to keep brushing your hair. As luck would have it, brushing is the wrong thing to do. It brings in more air and more humidity (especially on rainy days) and leaves hair even frizzier. For a better result, use some kind of texturizing cream or even conditioner when you brush, to keep hair strands smooth. And if you're really, honestly having an unbelievably bad hair day, go to the salon for a blowout.

Perhaps you're having a bad hair day simply because you're growing out an old cut, or maybe you didn't have the time to dry (or wash) your hair properly. If so, think of it as an opportunity to use some great hair accessories. Getting the hair out of the way, unless you have time to restyle it completely, is the best solution. Headbands, barrettes, a little impromptu updo with a stick are all chic camouflage for unhappy hair.

GROWING OUT A CUT

We get a lot of new clients looking for style changes in November—everyone wants to look their best for the holidays. Unfortunately it's not possible to erase a previous cut entirely unless you are willing to go *very* short. It's likely you'll have to spend some time in a transitional phase, growing out your existing cut.

Paradoxically, growing out a cut means more frequent haircuts. The idea is to get the layers to catch up with the ends as quickly as possible. As the layers grow, you trim the longest strands the most, cutting just enough off the shortest layers to keep the hair looking healthy. Also, because growing out hair involves awkward stages where there is no coherent style, more frequent cuts keep it neat and chic instead of wayward and out of control.

Talk to your stylist about the shape you'd like to coax your hair into as it

IF YOU HAVE A CASE OF NOVEMBER BLAHS, **ADD AN UNEXPECTED TOUCH OF COLOR TO YOUR WARDROBE—** A SPICY, ENERGIZING CORAL OR A DELICIOUS PALE BLUE.

7

IN THE COLDER MONTHS, **SUNGLASSES PROTECT YOUR EYES FROM THE WIND.** CHOOSE A PAIR WITH LENSES IN A LIGHT SHADE.

8

SCHEDULE YOUR SPRING VACATION RIGHT NOW. BUY NONREFUNDABLE PLANE TICKETS TO MAKE SURE YOU TAKE THE TIME TO GO OFF AND RELAX.

9

10 GET A HANDS-FREE, CORDLESS TELEPHONE WITH A HEADSET. HOLDING THE RECEIVER TO YOUR EAR IS SO TWENTIETH-CENTURY.

11 KEEP YOUR HOME FRESHLY SCENTED WITH AROMATIC WOODEN BALLS INSTEAD OF A POTPOURRI. NO MORE DUSTY ROSE PETALS LINGERING IN A BOWL.

12 BUY AN EXOTIC COOKBOOK AND COOK YOUR WAY THROUGH IT.

grows: A game plan is essential. So many women view the growing-out process as a period of inevitable awkwardness, when it really should be about the evolution of a style. You may end up surprising yourself with a length you love and want to keep, even though it isn't what you originally had in mind.

HAIR ORNAMENTS AND ACCESSORIES

Hair accessories (and styling products) are godsends when you are growing out your hair; of course, chic women use them to great effect no matter what the state of their hairstyle. The most important thing to remember about any hair accessory is that, above all, it needs to be functional. It's a stylish way of enhancing the look of your hair. I prefer hair accessories that have openings or cutouts to allow the hair to shine through.

HEADBANDS A headband is great for getting the hair off the face. It is especially practical for office work, when hair may tend to fall in your eyes while you're working. There are many stylish ones in all types of great materials and colors. As with barrettes, you'll want to experiment.

* **SOFT HEADBANDS** (complete circles, usually with elastic that goes under the hair) work well if your hair is shoulder-length or longer. On short or very thin hair, they tend to slide off.
* **HARD HEADBANDS** (U-shaped) come in a variety of widths and work with most hairstyles. Modern ones are designed to be flexible and adjustable, making them more comfortable than the old-fashioned ones.

RIGHT: A WHIMSICAL HEADBAND WILL KEEP BOTH YOU IN STYLE AND YOUR HAIR OFF YOUR FACE.

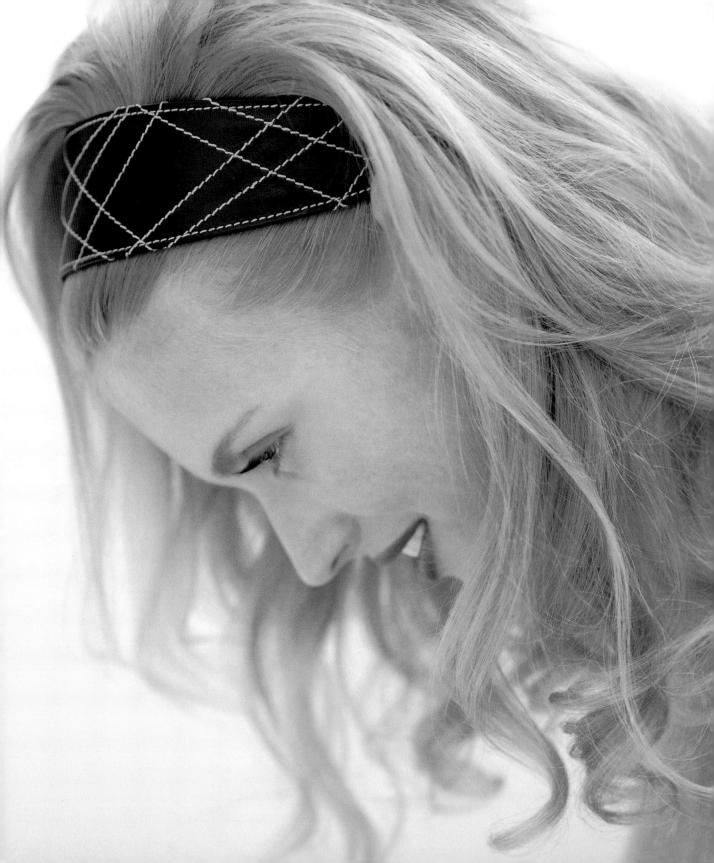

13

SPEND A QUIET EVENING AT HOME IN FRONT OF THE TELEVISION. INSTEAD OF EATING JUNK FOOD, THOUGH, INDULGE IN CAVIAR AND A GREAT BOTTLE OF CALIFORNIA CHARDONNAY.

14

DON'T HESITATE TO **REMOVE THE DESIGNER LABELS** FROM YOUR GARMENTS. FLAUNTING STATUS SYMBOLS IS NOT MODERN ANYMORE.

15

KEEP A HAND-SOFTENING CREAM NEXT TO YOUR COMPUTER. MASSAGE YOUR HANDS WITH CREAM WHILE WAITING FOR YOUR COMPUTER TO DOWNLOAD INFORMATION.

BARRETTES

* **I LOVE ELEGANT, SLEEK BARRETTES.** But a barrette that is only decorative is too fussy.

* **KEEP THE DESIGN OF YOUR BARRETTE SIMPLE,** but have fun with materials: Anything from grosgrain ribbon to leather to enamel to metal or even velvet can be fresh and pretty.

* **FOR EVENING,** choose a barrette that's a little more ornate, with maybe freshwater pearls or semi-precious stones. Make sure they complement the earrings and other jewelry you are wearing.

* **ROWS OF LITTLE BARRETTES CAN BE CUTE,** but don't get carried away. Two would work better than six.

* **IF A BARRETTE WON'T STAY IN YOUR HAIR,** don't try to get it to stay in place with gel or hairspray. Try another barrette.

PONYTAILS Whether or not you're growing your hair out, try a ponytail. Casual and fun, a ponytail quite literally gives you a pulled-together confidence.

* **PONYTAIL WRAPS ARE CHARMING,** but beware: They can be very frustrating the first time you try one. Always put hair in an elastic first, otherwise the wrap will eventually slide out.

* **IF YOUR HAIR TENDS TO BE FRIZZY,** run a little styling cream through it before you draw it back into a ponytail. After the elastic is in, make sure it's as sleek and perfect as you can get it. Then wrap on a coil or tie a ribbon around the elastic.

RIGHT: KEEP YOUR HAIRSTYLE SIMPLE WHEN YOU ARE WEARING A HAIR ORNAMENT. IT'S A FAST WAY TO GET A NEAT, MODERN LOOK.

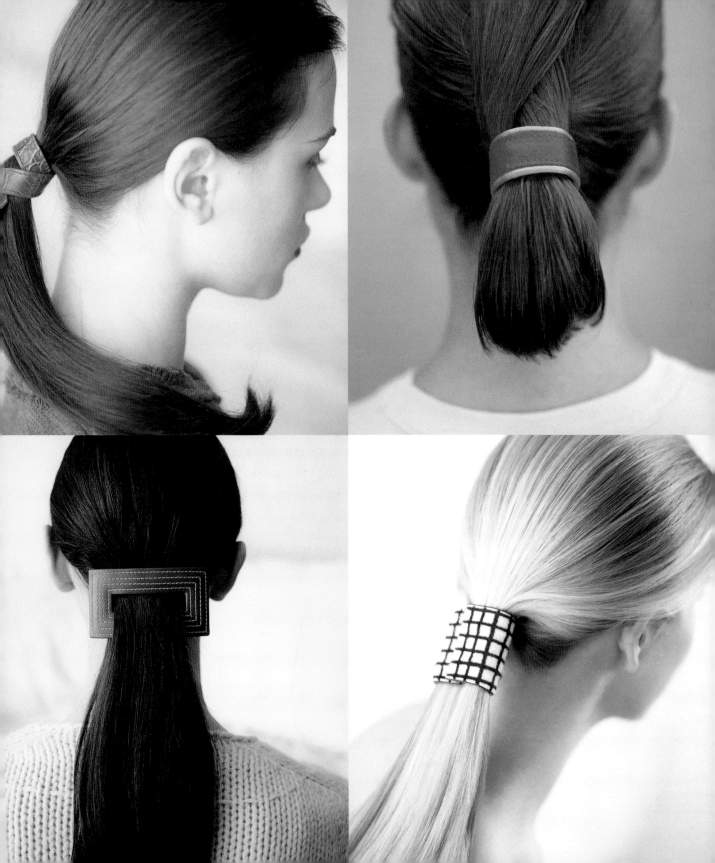

16

SEND HOLIDAY INVITATIONS OUT EARLY, SINCE EVERYONE'S CALENDAR FILLS UP FAST THIS TIME OF YEAR.

17

RINSE YOUR CONDITIONER THOROUGHLY UNDER THE SHOWER BY RUNNING A COMB THROUGH YOUR HAIR.

18

SCHEDULE A TEETH-WHITENING SESSION WITH YOUR DENTIST. IT'S ONE OF THE MOST AFFORDABLE AND EFFECTIVE WAYS TO BRIGHTEN YOUR FACE.

SHOPPING WITH STYLE

This year get a grip on your holiday shopping by starting early. And no dragging stuff around. Have everything shipped or sent to your home. You'll feel stylish. Decisive. Opinionated.

Pick a day or two, and clear your schedule. Get up, take a shower, and have a high-protein breakfast. Carry some dried fruit or something to keep you going in case you have to wait for lunch. Wear comfortable clothes that make you happy. Put your hair up in a ponytail (several of my clients tell me this makes them feel more efficient). While you're having breakfast, chart your course: Which stores will you cover? Whose gift will you buy where? Where to go first? Second? Where to have lunch? Be sure to make time for a coffee, mid-morning.

* **ENLIST THE HELP OF SALESPEOPLE.** Better yet, call beforehand and set up an appointment with someone who knows what you need.
* **HAVE THE STORES SEND THE PACKAGES** if that's more convenient, or, if you shop in a mall, have the clerks save the packages behind the desk, and then pick everything up on your way out (be sure to make a note of everything you bought and where to go back for them).
* **HAVE THINGS GIFT-WRAPPED** unless you really love doing it yourself, and customize the wrapping later with a glorious ribbon, a fantastic card, or little chocolates to attach to the bow, something that says, "I took time with this, because I love you."
* **BE RESOLUTELY CHEERFUL** with everyone you encounter—salespeople, wrappers, fellow shoppers. Your upbeat attitude will fortify overwhelmed store employees.
* **IF YOU GET TIRED,** have a refreshment and sit for a minute.
* **THE DAY OF SHOPPING** should never end with something strenuous. A bath or a massage is about the right speed. Or treat yourself to an early dinner out, at a very low-key spot.

GIVING GREAT GIFTS

As if life in November wasn't complicated enough, you have to steal from your busy schedule a couple of days at the end of the month to begin your holiday shopping. If you postpone it until next month, you are sure to turn what could be a pleasurable experience into a strenuous marathon. But you are faced with a nagging paradox: The only way to find the perfect present for everyone is to rush around town as slowly as you can.

Shopping early for gifts allows you to be more creative. You have enough time to order a gift from a craftsman or an artist. You can have linen monogrammed and stationery engraved. You can send for something from abroad. Or you can make a gift yourself by hand.

* THINK PRICELESS. A rare bottle of wine instead of a case of Bordeaux or champagne. When acquaintances send me a carefully selected bottle, to share with me their favorite vintage, I know they value my friendship. A first edition of Colette's *Chéri* sends the same message.

* THINK BIG. A jeroboam of champagne, a huge bouquet of French tulips, an oversized jar of perfumed body cream, even a huge beach towel or a large weekend bag are so much fun to receive. It's all about a grand gesture.

* THINK HEALTHY. Send a gift packed with vitamins, a huge basket of clementines, or a box of pomegranates. The more exotic, the better.

* THINK BACK. Is there a running joke between you and the person you are shopping for that would suggest a present? A gift that makes the recipient laugh is always a fabulous gift. Does any particular music suggest a time you spent together? Do you have a great picture of the two of you? Put it in a gorgeous frame or a photo album.

* THINK CASH. How about a scholarship for a stepdaughter, a godchild, or for an adult who wants to go back to school?

* THINK EXTRAVAGENT. A round-trip ticket to Paris for two.

* THINK CUDDLY. The best gift I ever got was a chocolate Labrador named Jessie. She was full of love and compassion and woke me up with kisses every morning. Everyone who saw her felt instantly more relaxed and happy.

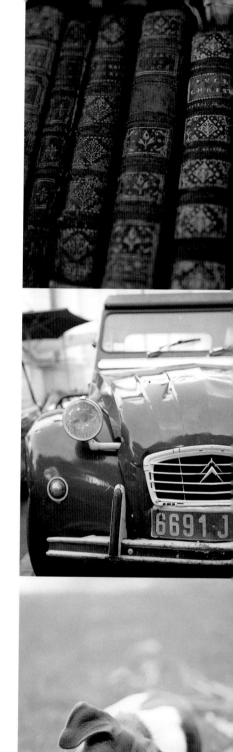

19

CENTRAL HEATING CAN BE DEHYDRATING. **KEEP A CARAFE OF WATER ON YOUR BEDSIDE TABLE** AND DRINK A GLASS AS SOON AS YOU WAKE UP.

20

DON'T OVERPLUCK YOUR EYEBROWS BETWEEN PROFESSIONAL SHAPINGS. IT MAKES YOUR FACE LOOK OUT OF BALANCE.

21

A woman is closest to being naked when she is well-dressed.

—COCO CHANEL

HOLIDAY CORRESPONDENCE

Holiday cards should arrive by the second week in December. Address and inscribe them all in November and relax. Cards are a charming, wonderful way to make—and maintain—a personal connection. It amazes me how many people simply type up a (lengthy) summation of their various movements and achievements during the year, barely bothering to sign it, and send it everywhere. What's more important, where you went on vacation, or how you feel about the friend you're writing to?

Cards should be simple, direct, and handwritten. A photo is a great thing to include. I especially love black-and-white photographs, but color can be charming, as can artwork—your own, your child's, or just a favorite image. A friend of mine always sketches his Christmas cards, and I have collected them all. When the card is personal, the message needn't be long, but it should be meaningful. Even something as simple as "We've got to see more of each other next year!" is better, to me, than a mind-numbing list of family activities.

Use old-style (thick, textural) paper. Choose rich colors. Ribbons are always wonderful. Imagination is everything. I usually write my cards over the course of several weeks, so I don't end up repeating the same message over and over.

RIGHT: THERE'S NO EXCUSE FOR BORING STATIONERY; THE PAPER, PENS, AND STAMPS YOU USE ALL SAY SOMETHING ABOUT YOUR STYLE.

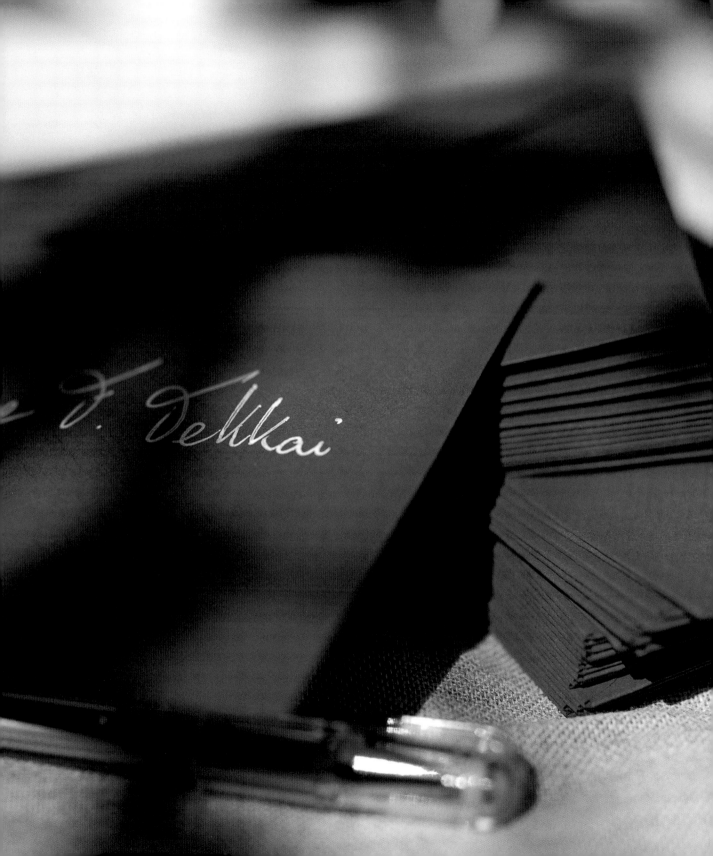

22

IT'S NOT TOO EARLY TO **START COLLECTING UNUSUAL PAPERS** FOR WRAPPING HOLIDAY GIFTS, SUCH AS POSTERS, OLD MAPS, OR FOREIGN NEWSPAPERS.

23

BUY THREE LIPSTICKS OF THE SAME COLOR. THE FIRST TUBE NEVER LEAVES YOUR DRESSING TABLE, THE SECOND STAYS IN YOUR COSMETICS BAG, WHILE THE THIRD TRAVELS WITH YOU IN YOUR CAR.

24

APPLY FOUNDATION EVENLY WITH A SPONGE OR A BRUSH, NOT WITH YOUR FINGERS. NO EXCEPTIONS. PERIOD.

IMPROMPTU SOCIALIZING

Though evening is the designated time for stylish get-togethers, some of the most stimulating conversations and some of the most creative networking take place during the day. You meet new people all the time, and if you have a curious mind and an open attitude you can have as much fun from nine to five as you do after hours.

Often, you meet people professionally, and there is an instant chemistry. If the circumstances were different, you would become friends. Sometimes, on impulse, as you say good-bye, you make plans to socialize, have lunch, visit on the weekend, go to a show or a sport event. You both know it might never happen (it probably won't, since we all are too busy) but the intention is sincere. This is what I call vicarious socializing, brief but exciting.

To get the most from these chance encounters, try the following:

* **DON'T LEAVE YOUR HOUSE WEARING** items that make you feel awkward, like a sweater that itches or badly scuffed shoes. There is nothing worse than misrepresenting yourself in public.
* **DON'T STRUGGLE TO BELONG.** Never adopt a look, like big hair or extra-long nails, just because it's the uniform where you work or live. Your time is better spent with people whose taste complements your own.
* **DON'T BE UNDULY IMPRESSED BY** folks who are more successful than you. Instead, be grateful: Unlike them, you will not be judged by your latest success or failure.
* **DON'T BE UNDULY IMPRESSED BY** blondes with va-va-voom figures: Behind their back, they are called bimbos.
* **DON'T BE UNDULY IMPRESSED BY** people who are better educated than you: Ask them about their lives, and they'll think you are very smart indeed.

At the salon, my clients are eager to socialize, too. They talk about everything: baseball, restaurants, Broadway shows. They share tips on which films to see and which vacation spots to try. Getting your highlights or your manicure is the next best thing to sitting at a terrace café and chatting with friends. And swaddled in a loose robe with damp hair falling around their ears, all my clients are equals.

Even people who've seen it all and done it all want to share ideas with me and other women in the salon.

Socialites are surprisingly friendly: Ann Bass, Nan Kempner, Mica Ertungun, Carol Petri. They don't have to try, which is refreshing. They are likely to come for a haircut and walk out of the salon with wet hair, because they have an appointment or they hate to fuss over details.

The most relaxed are the stage actresses who know how to handle the attention they create. They have guts; they are sexy; they are good looking. And they are not afraid to confront the public. With them, I chat about kids, schools, nutrition, relationships, diets—life, in other words.

Life? It's a big party.

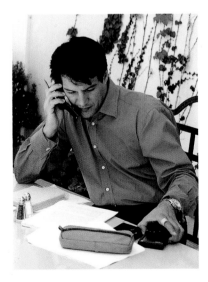

CHECK YOUR PASSPORT TO MAKE SURE IT ISN'T ABOUT TO EXPIRE. IT'S EASIER TO RENEW A PASSPORT THAN TO ORDER A NEW ONE.

25

TO EASE YOUR NERVES, **CONSIDER GIVING UP CAFFEINE OVER THE HOLIDAYS.** HOW ABOUT DRINKING HERBAL TEA INSTEAD? VERVAIN IS PARTICULARLY SOOTHING.

26

FIND A GOOD SALON-FORMULA SHAMPOO. YOUR HAIR NEEDS MORE PAMPERING IN WINTER, AND THE RIGHT PRODUCT MAKES ALL THE DIFFERENCE

27

28 BUY A FOUNTAIN PEN FOR
ADDRESSING HOLIDAY CARDS.

29 NEVER PRESS YOUR DINNER
GUESTS TO TAKE SECONDS.
YOU ARE NOT THEIR MOM.

30 BUY LUXURIOUS CASHMERE
SOCKS TO WEAR WITH YOUR
SNOW BOOTS.

KEEPING WARM

Winter country dressing is less high-tech than dressing for the ski slopes, with lots of layers that are both practical and stylish. The contrast between different textures and colors comes more into play: great boots in leather or suede—or tough rubber Wellingtons if it's slushy and mild—jeans or corduroys, car-length coats like Barbours, in oilcloth or leather, or even sheepskin.

Men and women alike look fantastic in this kind of dressing. Silk under-wear, worn under a great turtleneck in cashmere or wool, is sure to keep you warm. Think about wonderful fabrics and fibers: Irish wool, boiled wool, or the thick wool that French sailor's sweaters are made of. Think about subtle colors: oatmeal, chocolate brown, anthracite gray. Always bring extra pairs of thick cashmere socks and at least two great scarves. And never, ever, forget your hat.

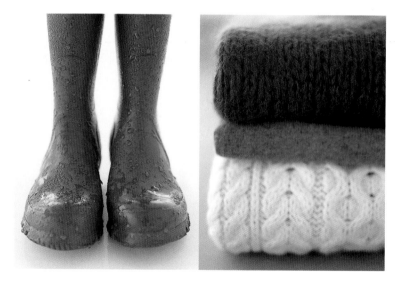

RIGHT: A SOFT KNITTED AFGHAN IS WINTER'S MOST
LUXURIOUS WAY TO KEEP THE COLD AT BAY.

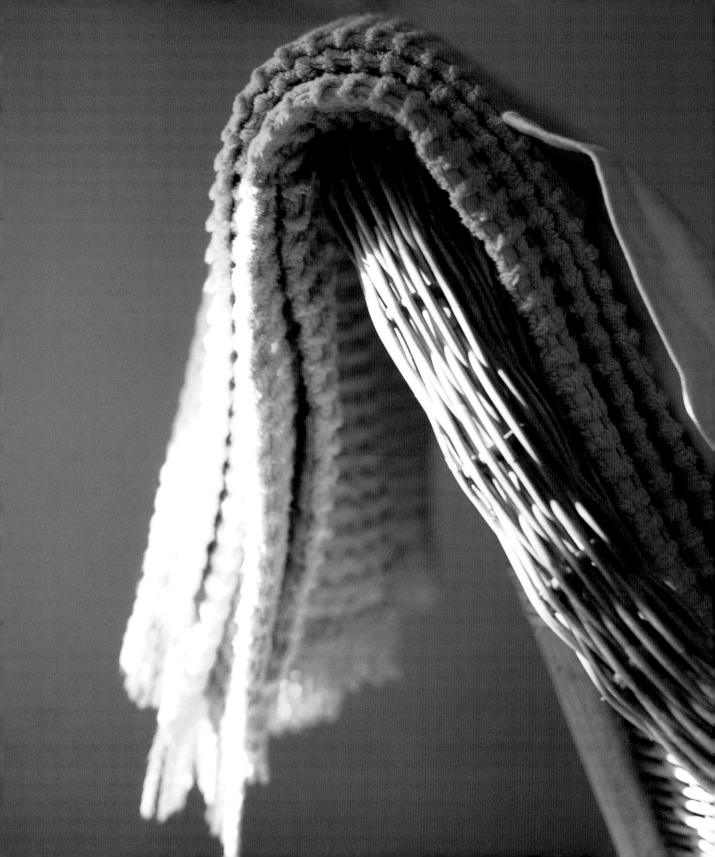

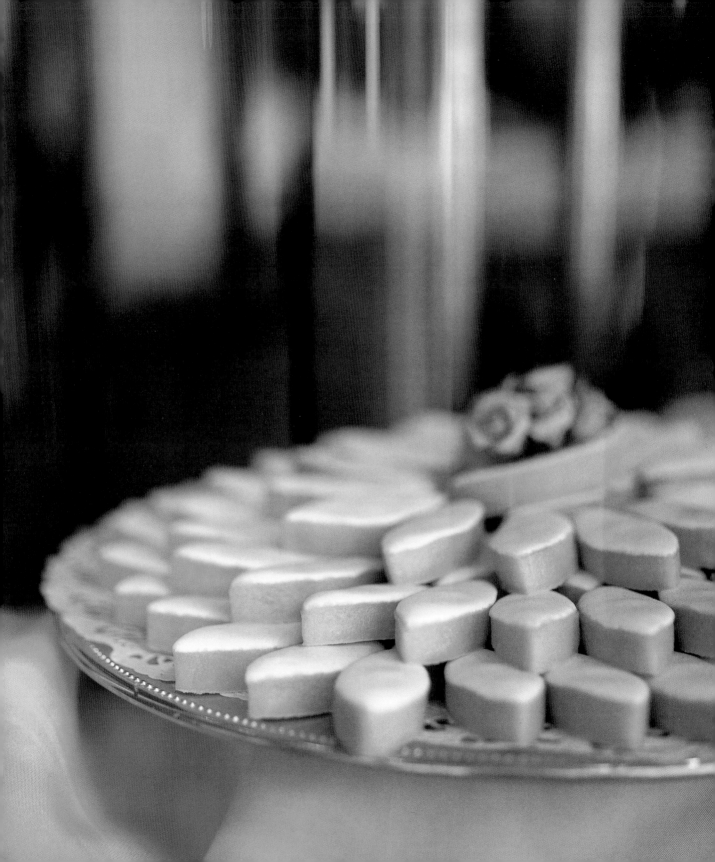

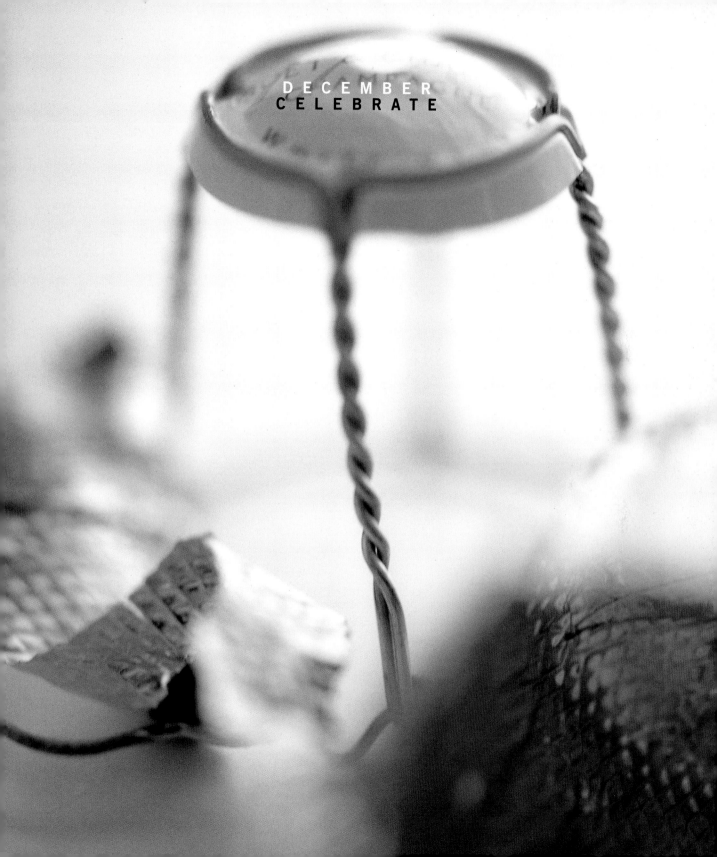

DECEMBER
CELEBRATE

PRIORITIZE. DON'T TRY TO ACCOMPLISH TOO MUCH AT THIS TIME OF THE YEAR.

POSTPONE WHAT'S NOT ESSENTIAL TILL NEXT YEAR.

CONTRIBUTE TO CHARITIES THAT BENEFIT NEEDY CHILDREN.

As the end of the year approaches, we all instinctively find our way back home—whether literally or figuratively. The parties are just as numerous and upbeat as they were in November, but somehow the mood grows more intimate. When going out, you still dress with flair, even panache, but you are not trying to impress everyone. December is a time to be comfortable with who you are, to reach out for real friends, and to remember loved ones.

During the holidays, be generous with people in need, but avoid schmaltzy sentimentality, forced smiles, and sugar-coated wishes—'tis the season to be sincere. Nothing is more tasteless than pretending to be merry at a boring Christmas function, or spending too much money on a pointless gift for an acquaintance who has everything. Whenever I feel anxious instead of excited at this time of the year, I know what to do: I give something special to someone who either needs it or will adore it.

RIGHT: BE ORIGINAL. LOOK FOR BEAUTIFUL RIBBONS AND PRINTED PAPERS ALL YEAR LONG TO MAKE YOUR HOLIDAY GIFTS UNIQUE.

DESIGN YOUR OWN GREETING CARDS, BUT DON'T USE THOSE TACKY DRUGSTORE PHOTO CONTRAPTIONS.

A SPECIAL HOLIDAY DESSERT: WHOLE PEARS PEELED, BLANCHED, AND BROWNED IN BUTTER UNTIL LIGHTLY GLAZED. SERVE IN A GLASS, WITH VANILLA ICE CREAM.

Everybody wants to be Cary Grant. Even I want to be Cary Grant.

—CARY GRANT

It's best to channel the energy of the holidays into simple pleasures, like making your own greeting cards or decorations, helping a neighbor trim a tree, spending time on the phone with relatives, digging out Julia Child's recipe for gâteau Victoire au chocolat, or buying handmade gifts from the people who made them.

I also think that it's a good time to ask artists or talented friends to help you create a special holiday event. Organize a private concert in your living room during which local musicians perform for a small audience; you provide the food, they provide the entertainment, and your guests provide the applause. Or arrange for an exhibition of the work of a painter or sculptor you admire even though he or she is not yet famous. Or have a cake sale to make money for neighborhood kids. Practice a little grassroots philanthropy and I promise that you will feel more holiday cheer.

TRADITIONS

Traditions, family or otherwise, are the stuff great style is made of. Whether you spend the holidays skiing in Sun Valley, or sunning on the beach in Hawaii, or simply at home, create holiday rituals that you repeat year in and year out.

An older couple I know has an antique, child-size electric train that they set up every year as the holiday approaches, delighting their friends and grandchildren. Another friend is famous for her incredible arrangements of all-white flowers in silver cups. I myself love to cook for friends during the holidays and make quite an impression when I throw together on short notice a roasted pheasant with braised endives, or pears browned in butter, slightly glazed, served in a glass, with some ice cream on top.

In Provence, as in many parts of the world, holiday traditions center around food. As a child I looked forward each year to the orgy of sweets known as the Thirteen Desserts, in memory of Christ and the twelve apostles. On cold, dark afternoons, we'd drink homemade hot chocolate and enjoy it with homemade cookies, another Provençal tradition. In the evenings, the holiday drink is *vin d'orange,* hot red wine mixed in a large pot with herbs and spices, then served in glass mugs or wonderful old teacups, each one a different pattern. And for Christmas dinner, there was always a goose with roasted potatoes. Hard cider was served as well as a few very good bottles of local wine.

Though we all love exotic preparations for the holidays, simple fare is often just as fun. For me, improvisation is always the main ingredient in any recipe. I cook the way I cut hair: I am inspired by the people I am with. If they like to eat, I rise to the occasion and produce a fabulous meal. The following are some of my favorite easy recipes for impromptu get-togethers with close friends and family.

* **Tian de pommes de terre:** baked potatoes cubed and cooked in the oven in a fresh tomato purée with olive oil, garlic, and Provençal herbs. If you like, add some grated cheese and onions to the mix.
* **Macédoine de legumes:** a cold salad of cooked potatoes and baby carrots cut in small cubes tossed with tiny green peas, chopped parsley (lots of it), and a light homemade mayonnaise dressing.
* **Brouillade aux cêpes:** scrambled eggs, cooked slowly in a double-boiler with sautéed wild mushrooms. Also delicious: scrambled eggs with fresh, skinless tomatoes and basil leaves.
* **Blanquette de veau:** Veal stew in a light lemony white sauce, served with rice.
* **Green salad with warm goat cheese.**

On December 24, I like to cook a more elaborate feast, like a goose stuffed with pineapple and oranges. We usually start the evening with champagne, then serve Sauterne wine to go with the foie gras on toast. Oysters, served with vinegar and lemon slices are also on the menu, and bottles of white Riesling or Sancerre are never far away.

HONEY SPICE CAKE

This is my mother's recipe; it's wonderful with a cup of tea.

½ cup sugar
2 cups all-purpose flour
1 teaspoon baking soda
1 teaspoon apple pie spice
2 teaspoons aniseed
½ teaspoon ground cinnamon
½ teaspoon ground cloves
1 cup scalded milk
2 teaspoons rum
2 teaspoons honey

Combine the sugar, flour, baking soda, apple pie spice, aniseed, cinnamon, and cloves in a large bowl and mix well. In a measuring cup combine the milk with the rum and honey. Add to the flour mixture and stir with a wooden spoon until smooth. Cover and let stand overnight at room temperature.

The next day, preheat the oven to 350°F. Grease a large loaf pan, then line the bottom with parchment paper and grease the paper. Spoon the batter into the prepared pan; it should not be more than half full. Cover with foil and bake for 45 minutes. Cool completely in the pan before slicing.

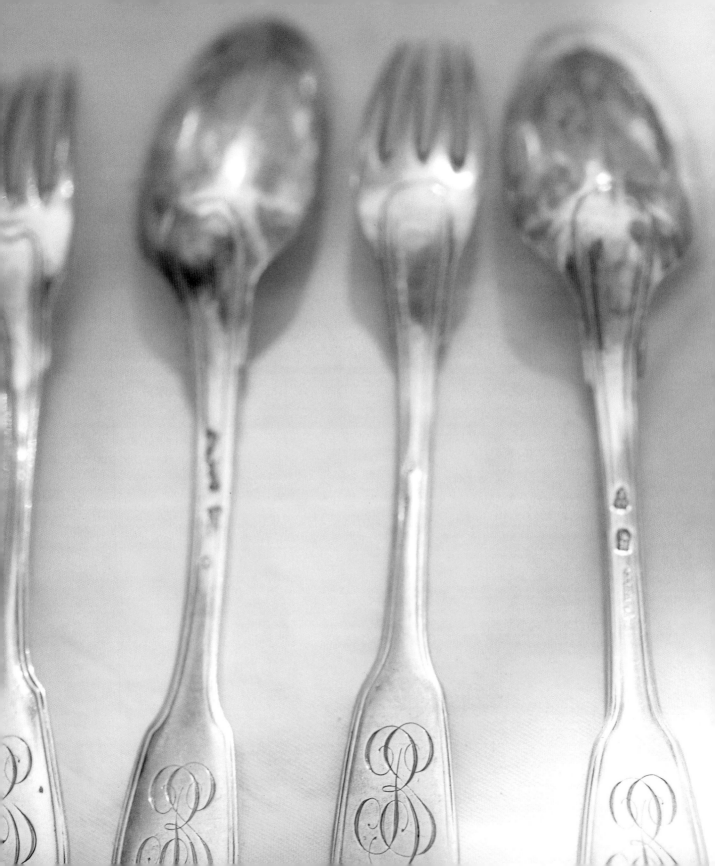

THE STYLISH HOLIDAY HOME

The thing that makes holiday traditions so enjoyable is the anticipation—you know what's going to happen, and you've been waiting for it all year. It's just the way a theme for a party gets people in the mood; it's the thinking about it beforehand that makes it all the more fun.

As the host, you can be very deliberate in your style, and your friends and family will remember your special efforts year after year. Develop a holiday signature: maybe it's a great ginger cookie recipe that you pull out only once a year, or the fact that you fill the house with white narcissus. Or, host a party each year at which only a particular kind of champagne is served, or, like many English families, hard cider.

Fill your home with holiday colors, sounds, and scents: music, candles, ribbons, wrapping paper, baskets of fruits, sweets in bowls, candies in jars. Though red and green is the traditional color scheme, you don't have to feel obliged to use both colors at once—or either!

* Try a white holiday with crystal, silver, palest blue—think of the color of pearls and snow.
* Natural colors are surprisingly warm and upbeat: pastels, kraft paper, beeswax candles, bouquets of holly here and there to establish the holiday theme.
* Decorate your table with handwritten place cards.
* Set a little box with a special gift next to each place setting.
* Make *papillotes* for the table—delicious sweets, chocolates, marzipan, or candied fruits rolled in layers of pretty, crinkly papers with the ends twisted, like butterflies.
* Give the children their own party beforehand, with their own decor, so they won't be hungry and cranky when the grown-ups are ready to sit down for dinner.

TIPS FOR A RELAXED HOLIDAY PARTY

Don't try to do it all alone. Share the holiday spirit with your guests by asking them to help you: Get someone to open the oysters, someone else to empty the dishwasher, a third person to set the table, and so on. There is plenty to do for anyone eager to participate and break the ice: prepare appetizers, light the candles, put on the music, open the wine.

Give everyone who arrives early something to do, and something to eat and drink. This initiates the festivities even before the official party starts. Get the ball rolling ahead of schedule.

Begin anew as you celebrate the end of a great year.

HONE YOUR TABLE MANNERS: NEVER USE A STEEL KNIFE WITH FISH; USE A FLAT SILVER KNIFE INSTEAD.

GET A GREAT GLOSS TO ADD A LAYER OF SHINE TO YOUR FAVORITE LIPSTICK.

AVOID OVERINDULGING IN DRINK AT HOLIDAY WORK PARTIES—YOU'LL REGRET IT.

DINING OUT

My favorite holiday pastime, of course, is going out to eat with friends. I choose restaurants that fit the mood of the moment and the people I am with. Knowing how to select just the right place to eat is a skill as critical as knowing how to dress for a special occasion. My clients ask me almost as many questions about restaurants as they do about hair and makeup. It's not about knowing which are the new "in" spots with waiting lists a mile long and attitude to match; the key is choosing a spot that suits the company, offering just the right level of formality and sophistication in both food and atmosphere to make them feel at ease.

* **WITH FAMILY OR CHILDHOOD FRIENDS,** I opt for authentic French restaurants that serve regional cuisine. As a rule, French, Italian, and ethnic restaurants promote conviviality. If you are going out with your parents, in particular, stay away from stuffy eateries where everyone is afraid to use the wrong fork. Choose a less expensive place, order more dishes, and have fun.

* **WITH THE FASHIONABLE CROWD,** I am more likely to suggest the latest trendy bistro, or a sushi bar in an up-and-coming neighborhood. For trendsetters, seeing and being seen is more important than eating quietly. These places are usually very noisy, but never mind. The high decibel level seems only to add to the exhilarating mood.

* **WITH CLOSE FRIENDS,** I make reservations at a downtown brasserie where the food is a delicious mix of fancy Northern Italian cuisine and French bourgeois cooking. The scene is as lively and eclectic as the food, and it makes everyone feel younger. I am partial to places where the tiles, the walls, and the various surfaces are buffed, not glossy; people look both chic and scruffy, and I always make a mental note of what everyone's wearing.

RIGHT: EVEN IN THIS BUSIEST OF MONTHS
I TRY TO MAKE TIME FOR LUNCH WITH
FRIENDS ONCE OR TWICE A WEEK.

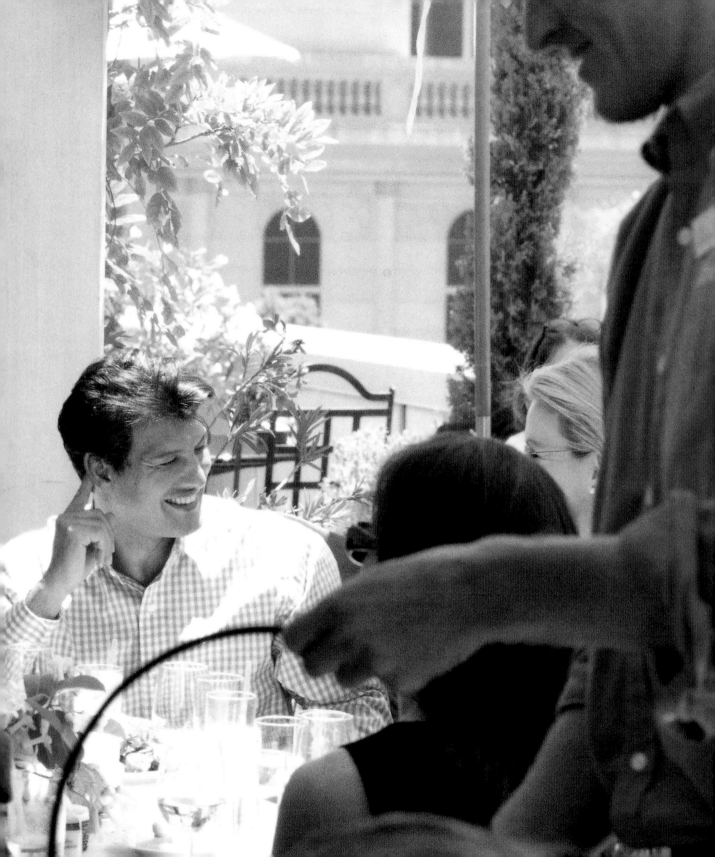

10

MAKE *PAPILLOTE* TABLE DECORATIONS. CUT 12 X 12-INCH SQUARES OF CRINKLY PAPER IN VARIOUS COLORS. LAYER TWO SQUARES AND ARRANGE THREE OR FOUR CHOCOLATES, MARZIPAN, OR CANDIED FRUITS IN THE MIDDLE. ROLL INTO A TUBE THEN TWIST THE ENDS.

11

BUY A CD OF FRENCH SINGING LEGEND GEORGES BRASSENS. HIS WARM BARITONE AND LAID-BACK GUITAR PLAYING WILL PUT YOU IN THE MOOD FOR AN EASYGOING EVENING WITH GOOD FRIENDS.

12

INSTEAD OF ORDERING A TURKEY FOR CHRISTMAS DINNER, **ORDER A GOOSE.** STUFF IT WITH BRIOCHE, PRUNES, AND CHESTNUTS. SERVE WITH ROASTED POTATOES.

HOW TO READ A MENU

As important as choosing the right restaurant is knowing how to read its menu. In the minds of many people, fear of snooty waiters nearly rivals the fear of public speaking. But there's no trick to getting good service if you observe good sense and common courtesy.

✳ **DON'T LET YOURSELF BE INTIMIDATED** by waiters or menus. If something on the menu is unfamiliar, ask questions until you are satisfied. If you have strong preferences, let the waiter know so he can guide you; only the staff knows if your least favorite ingredients are lurking in a sauce, and you won't find out if you don't ask. This doesn't make you a pain in the neck. On the contrary, it shows you are an attentive connoisseur.

✳ **ANTICIPATE WHAT YOU'LL BE DOING AFTER** your meal and order accordingly. Lunch is different from dinner. Think of what will give you energy or calm you down, depending on your schedule. Don't hesitate to order two appetizers if you don't want to be slowed down by getting filled up.

✳ **NEVER ORDER TWO** consecutive dishes featuring fish or meat. Vary your choices so you can savor each.

✳ **BETWEEN FRIENDS,** it's nice to discuss what each person is ordering. It's a good way to stimulate your imagination and your appetite.

✳ **DON'T SHARE MAIN COURSES;** you'll confuse your taste buds with lots of different flavors. Eat only what's on your plate in order to enjoy the various flavors the chef has carefully assembled.

✳ **EAT YOUR SALAD AFTER,** not before, the main course to aid digestion.

✳ **DON'T FEEL OBLIGED TO SHARE A DESSERT.** In fact, it's quite sexy to freely indulge your sweet tooth. And remember: a small rich pastry may have fewer calories than a huge slice of "low-fat" cake or even a fruit dessert.

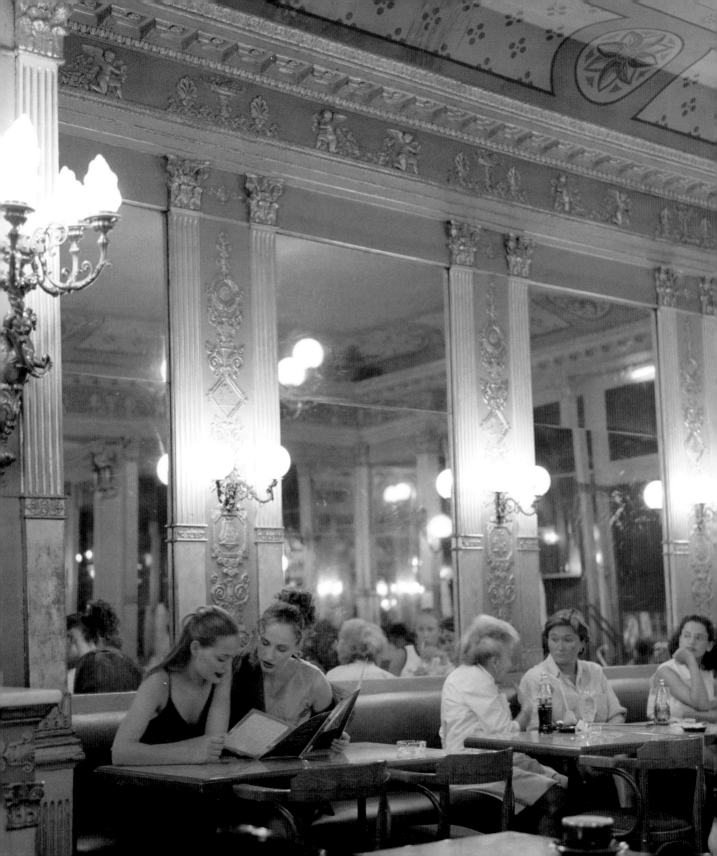

LOOKING
AS FABULOUS AS YOU FEEL

In December, mood is everything, and celebrating in comfort is key to feeling merry. Dress in colors that are both cozy and serene: jewel tones, deep burgundy, dark blues, muted green, chocolate, black, rich ochers or yellows. If you like red, this is the time to wear it. Favor velvets, silk, and warm yet weightless fabrics that envelop you like a cocoon. Combine textures and colors that reflect the light with a soft glow rather than a harsh shine.

When getting dressed for a holiday party, pamper your senses and you will uplift your spirit. The clothes you choose should be quietly luxurious. Wear a velvet skirt with suede boots. Team a pastel silk skirt with a cashmere shawl. Rediscover Scottish plaids. Find one simple jewel, and wear it all through the season. Throw a big pale blue or dark green coat over everything. Your festive outfits need to make you feel confident, attractive, and charming, without ever distracting from your personality.

* **BE ELEGANT** but do not show off.
* **BE CUDDLY.** If the fabrics have a wonderful texture, you'll feel contented and cheerful wearing them, and people will want to touch and hug you.
* **ADD A TOUCH OF COLOR.** Even if everything else is black, it always looks right. A wrap in a wonderful color takes any ensemble to a new level. Just be sure the clothes you're wearing with it aren't so colorful themselves that they fight each other.
* **FOR NEW YEAR'S EVE** black-tie parties, shift to lighter colors. Wear a silk suit or a strapless dress in light gray or pale blue, for example.
* **SHOW A LITTLE SKIN,** at the shoulders, perhaps, or legs. It is incredibly appealing, especially in the winter. But wildly plunging necklines or micro-mini skirts have a desperate quality that's decidedly unfestive.

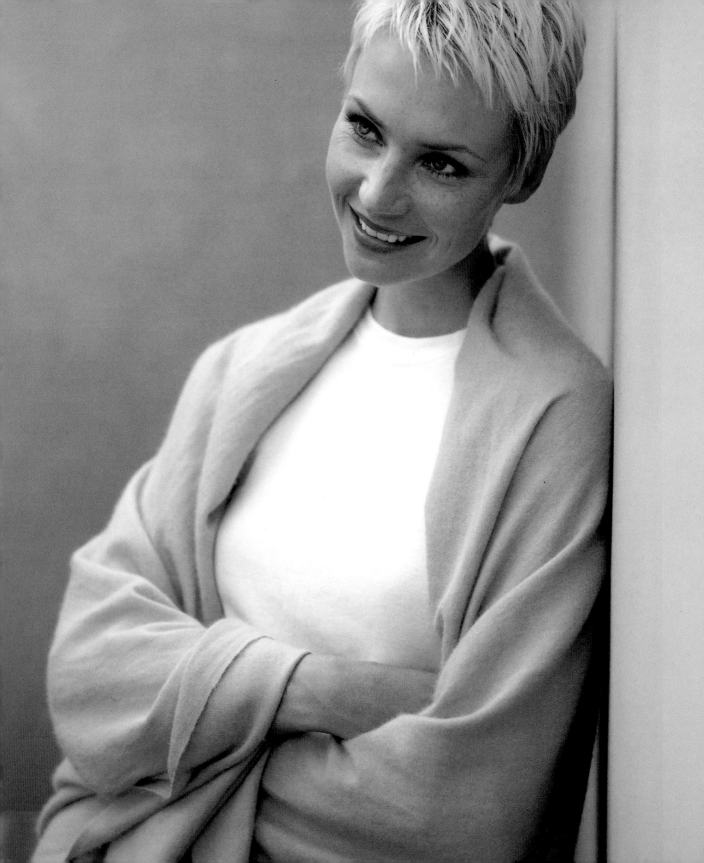

16 TOO MUCH TO DO? **DON'T WORRY ABOUT EVERYTHING AT ONCE.** JUST CONCENTRATE ON THE NEXT THING ON YOUR SCHEDULE.

17 GIVE SOMEONE ON YOUR LIST A SET OF REALLY GOOD HAIR BRUSHES.

18 **FILL HIS BIG WINTER BOOTS** WITH SMALL GIFTS AS THE FRENCH DO.

* **FOR AFTERNOON PARTIES,** go wintry, casual chic: corduroy or tweed suits for men, mid-calf velvet or cashmere dresses for women.

* **GIVE YOUR KIDS SOMETHING TO REMEMBER.** Insist they wear party clothes bought for the occasion, like plaid dresses for girls, dark velvet suits for boys.

* **DAY OR NIGHT,** a turtleneck in cashmere covers a multitude of worries, and focuses the attention on your face.

* **WEAR JEWELRY PIECES** that sparkle like snow: rhinestones or pearls.

* **KEEP MAKEUP SIMPLE,** not gaudy. Try a soft red or wine-colored lipstick rather than a hot red; use a gloss or a lip stain, perhaps.

* **A TOUCH OF SPARKLE,** over the eyes, for instance, or even with cream blush on the cheeks or mixed with lipstick on the lips, can be fun if your skin is in great condition and you're not wearing heavy makeup.

* **HAIR SHOULD BE RELAXED IN STYLE,** well conditioned, shiny. No hairspray (at least none that's visible).

* **A WISELY PLACED BARRETTE** or hair ribbon can make everything you wear more chic.

* **A FESTIVE BAG** with whimsical details of beads or embroidery is utterly stylish and appropriate.

* **HEELS ARE DEFINITELY DRESSED-UP,** but so are velvet or suede slippers.

* **HAVE A PEDICURE IN A COLOR THAT'S DELICIOUS.** Even if your toes don't show, beautifully done toes make you feel sensual.

RIGHT: AN ALTERNATIVE TO BOLD MAKEUP, SHIMMERY EYES AND PALE LIPS MAKE A FESTIVE FACE.

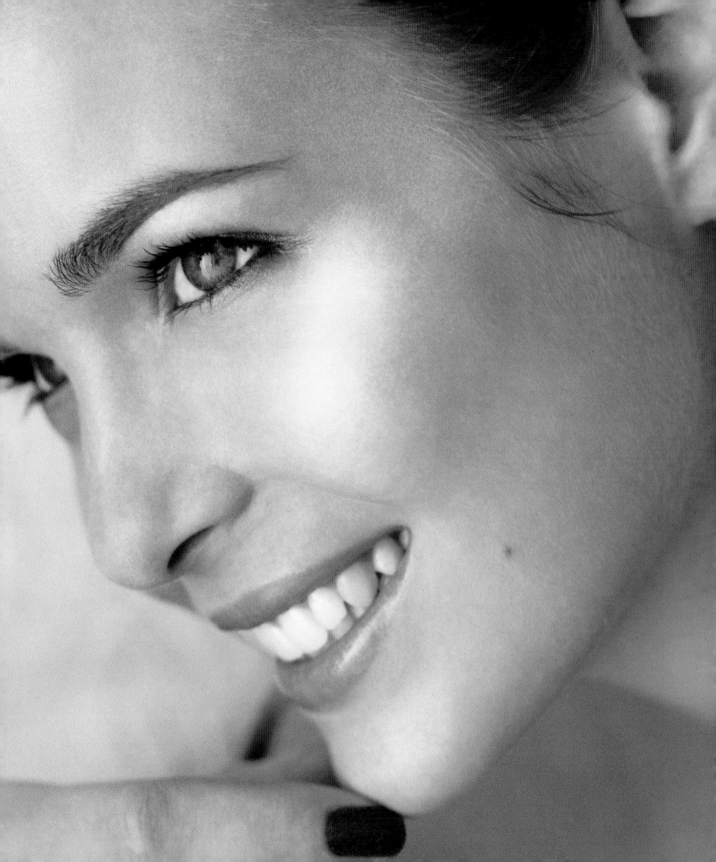

TIP FOR A HOST: MAKE SURE THAT YOU **TALK TO YOUR GUESTS ABOUT WHAT INTERESTS THEM,** NOT ABOUT WHAT INTERESTS YOU.

A THREE-STEP PARTY MAKEOVER: PUT YOUR HAIR UP, BRUSH ON SOME RED LIPSTICK, AND CLIP ON YOUR MOST FABULOUS EARRINGS.

GIVE A BUSY MOTHER A HUGE BOTTLE OF BUBBLE BATH TIED IN A PRETTY BATH MAT.

ENDING THE YEAR IN STYLE

A sure way to maintain a spirit of celebration is to take a little time off for yourself. I encourage clients to book massages, wraps, sea-salt scrubs—things that are not only relaxing, but also keep you in touch with your body. It's very easy, during the holidays, to find excuses for eating everything in sight and, in the process, jeopardize your physical and mental well-being.

Body treatments put things back into perspective, so you're less likely to abandon all your good fitness and eating habits. Eat more vegetables at every meal this month. Drink herbal tea if you're feeling hungry or cold, or simply in need of soothing. Get to the gym as often as possible; you can wrap the presents, answer calls, finish the cards later. Don't postpone getting back in shape till January. Get a head start on your New Year's resolutions. Enjoy the holidays by keeping everything on an even keel!

Of course everyone frets about gaining weight at this time of the year, but it's hardly the time to adopt a rigorous or strict regimen. Diets don't work, say the experts. So don't bother with some crazy diet that has you counting calories, ordering things like baked potatoes with squeezed lemon, or banishing half your refrigerator. For me, dieting is synonymous with eating well, eating good, good-for-you ingredients. If you do that instead of starving yourself, you will find your ideal weight and your ideal energy balance.

That said, it never hurts to avoid greasy food, canned food, and fast food. You should also try not to drink hard liquor while you're eating. Have a glass of red wine, instead. And at all costs, avoid having just a single big meal. You should ideally eat something every four hours, preferably smaller portions of very fresh food.

RIGHT: WHEN I HAVE TIME FOR MYSELF, I LOVE TO TAKE OFF IN A ROADSTER WITH THE TOP DOWN.

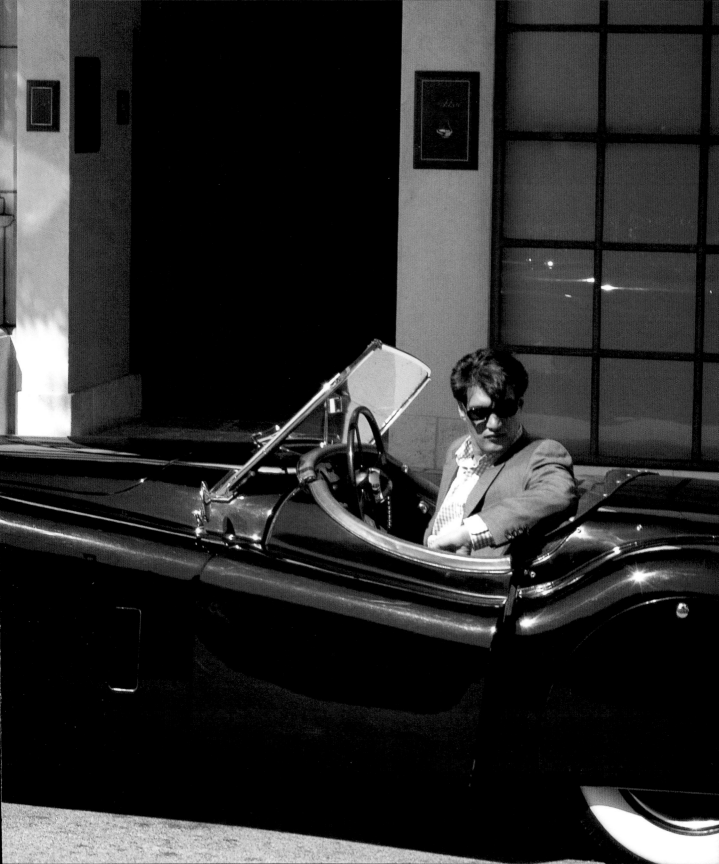

WINTER HAIR AND SCALP

Cold, dry, winter air, coupled with indoor heat and heat-based styling tools like blow-dryers, can leave your hair abused—frizzy, uncooperative, full of split ends, and lacking its usual healthy sheen. A dry scalp, though often exacerbated by the same conditions, involves different problems: Your head feels itchy; the skin under your hair feels tight. The frizziness is less on the ends and more at the roots. The treatments for these two related but different conditions are not the same.

A dry scalp needs the attention of a professional, someone able to assess the situation correctly. An itchy, flaking scalp can actually be a sign of too much oil; in other cases, it's the opposite. Scalp treatments, not conditioning treatments designed for the hair, but treatments specifically for the skin on your scalp, can be enormously helpful to people with very oily scalps, extremely dry scalps, or dandruff. They're best done at a salon, after a serious consultation. Last but not least, if your scalp feels and looks fine, and your hair's healthy, shiny, and bouncy, be suspicious of any stylist who tries to sell you on a scalp treatment.

Abused hair, on the other hand, is easier to diagnose, and generally should be treated with extra conditioning: Put on a hair mask and leave it on while you work out, for instance. Get a deep-conditioning treatment at a salon (good ones will involve a conditioning agent and some kind of heat, like a warm towel or even a hair dryer). And, after you've dried your hair, apply finishing cream to the ends until your hair is its soft, silky self once again.

RIGHT: WHEN YOU APPLY A HAIR MASK, BE SURE TO COMB IT ALL THE WAY THROUGH YOUR HAIR, FROM ROOTS TO ENDS.

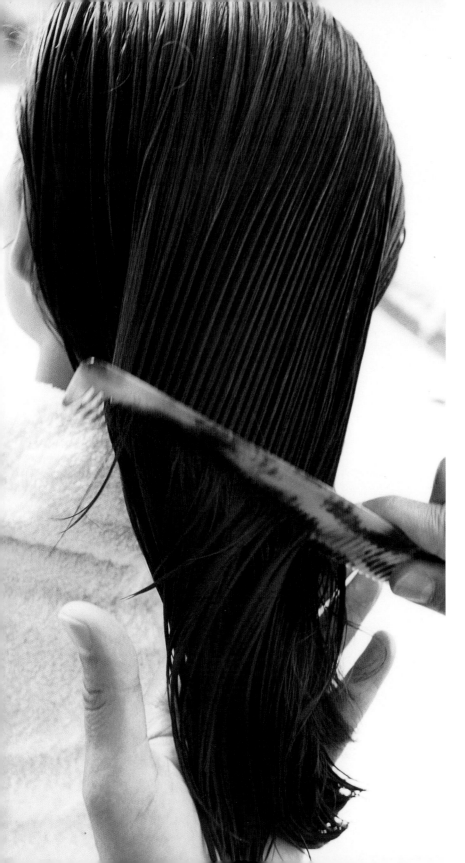

FIGHTING WINTER DRYNESS

In the wintertime, almost everyone's skin gets dry. So drink lots of water, and moisturize, moisturize, moisturize.

∗ USE A HUMIDIFIER in your bedroom and office.

∗ DON'T SPEND TOO MUCH TIME in hot baths or steam rooms; they seem like they would be the best treatments, when in fact, they're the worst. Hot water actually dries your skin, so keep baths short and lukewarm, unappealing as it sounds.

∗ TRY A RICHER FACIAL DAY CREAM formula than the one you normally use.

∗ FOR REALLY DRY, scaly skin, try one of the many creams with alphahydroxy acids. They were developed for extremely dry skin.

∗ GET A BODY MASSAGE OR WRAP with moisturizing oils.

NEW YEAR'S EVE FACE, SOPHISTICATED AND SEXY

It's tempting to be overzealous with makeup on this ultra-glamorous holiday. But think about your surroundings on New Year's: No matter where you are, there's going to be a lot of glitter and sparkle. Why try to compete? Go for an understated glamour that is both soft and sexy—an ideal way to mark the beginning of the new year. One way to achieve this is with a vibrant red mouth and a subtle shimmer on the eyes.

LIPS This sophisticated, sexy look is all about a vibrant, sensual mouth. The best way to draw attention to the lips is with the perfect red lipstick. Depending on your skin tone, your perfect red may be a brick with orange undertones, a ruby that's more blue, or a browner neutral red! To complement the elegance of the gold shadow (see below), choose a lipstick that's either deep red or a red with orange undertones. The lipstick should not be too metallic or shimmery for this sophisticated face. Apply a smooth, even coat over lip pencil for longer wear. Remember, red will draw attention to your lips so plan to touch up (always in the ladies' room) during the evening.

NAILS On the hands, use a very sheer color in the pale zone. With red lips, you'll be better off keeping hands subtle. For the toes, you can pick a bright red color, especially great for strappy, glittery party shoes.

EYES To complement a vibrant mouth, keep eyes simple. Be sure your brows are nicely shaped and groomed. Pluck any extraneous hairs (see page 207) and fill in as necessary with a brow pencil that matches your brow coloring. Choose a deep gold color or another subtle metallic for shadow, and with a brush, apply the shadow sheerly across the lid and up to the brow bone. Apply two coats of black mascara to finish the eyes.

CHEEKS Look for a blush in the pink family, with warm earthy undertones. Softly sweep your blush brush across your cheeks, lightly grazing the bridge of your nose, your forehead, and chin. The color should appear warm and balanced across your face.

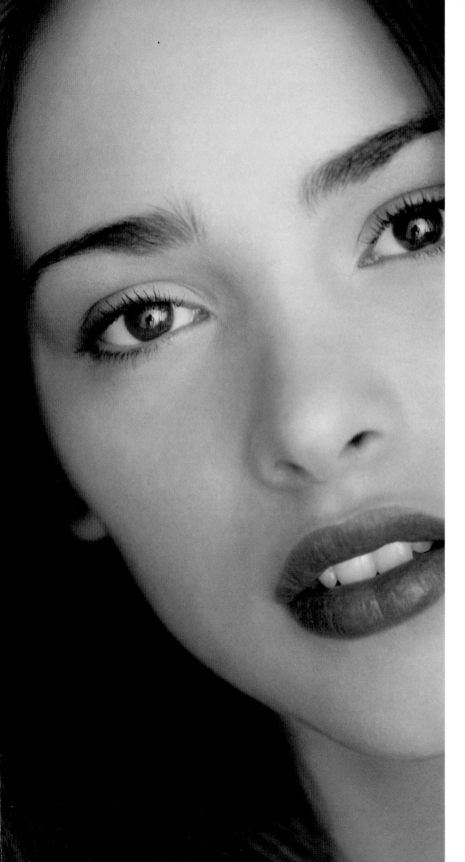

GETTING READY TO GO OUT SHOULD BE AS MUCH FUN AS POSSIBLE. **PUT SOME MUSIC ON WHILE YOU DRESS.** DON'T WAIT FOR THE LAST MINUTE TO GET IN A FESTIVE MOOD.

28

THOUGH IT'S COLD AND WINDY, **WALK WITH A LARGE, EASY STRIDE.** YOU'LL STAY WARMER, LOOK TALLER, AND HAVE MORE FUN. DON'T LET THE WEATHER CRAMP YOUR STYLE.

29

I know of only one duty, and that is to love.

—ALBERT CAMUS

30

REPEAT AFTER ME: "APPRE-CIATION, LOVE, HUMOR, AND PASSION ARE THE MAIN INGREDIENTS OF STYLE."

31

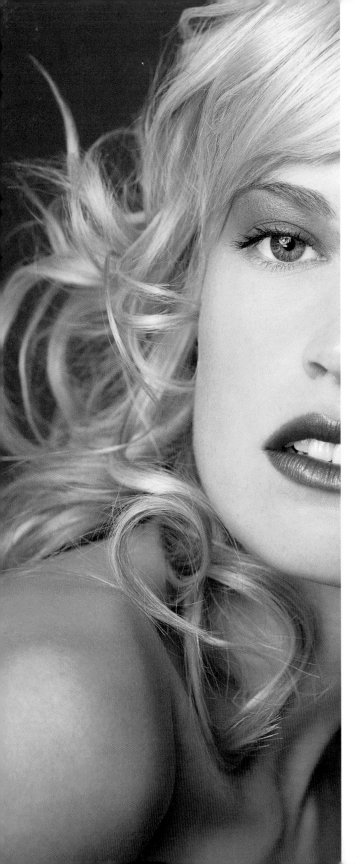

OVER-THE-TOP HAIR

Anything can happen when the clock strikes midnight on New Year's Eve. Be ready for the unexpected: Deck yourself to the nines and dare to do something extravagant with your hair. Even the most excessive hairstyle will simply look festive. Here are a few options.

USE A CURLING IRON on straight hair for a full head of romantically loose curls.

LET YOUR HAIR DOWN but clip bejeweled hair accessories in your wild coiffure.

SWEEP YOUR HAIR UP in a loose updo and secure your locks with large decorative hairpins or beautifully crafted ornamental clips.

GO FOR LOTS OF RINGLETS but twist them back and anchor them off your face with bobby pins.

OPT FOR SLEEK AND SEXY, using finishing cream to add luster to your hair. Let your straight and shiny do swing freely all night long.

KEEP IT BOUNCY AND EFFORTLESS, as if you did it yourself—even if you spent hours at the hair salon.

Whatever look you adopt, capture the spirit of the holidays by getting rid of your hairstyle inhibitions.

HAPPY NEW YEAR!

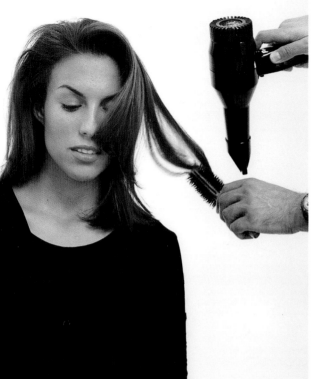

1 | 3
2 | 4

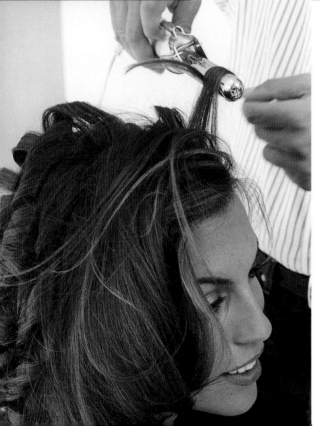

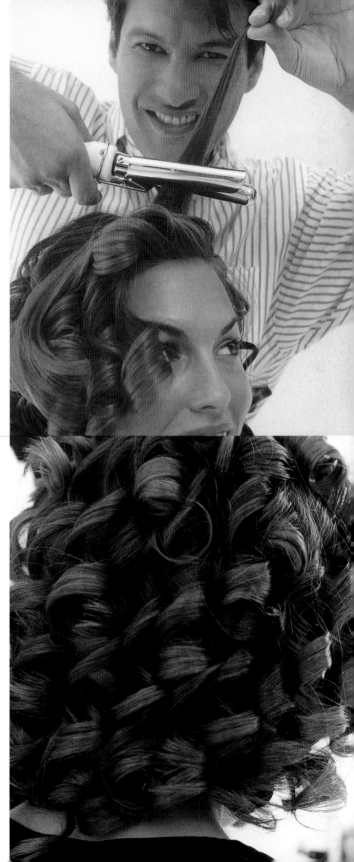

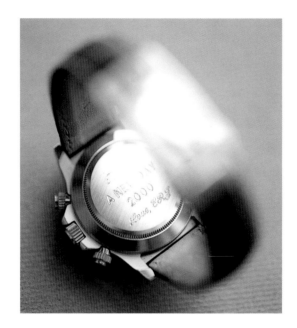